Problems in
Ophthalmology

Problems in Practice Series

PROBLEMS IN ARTHRITIS AND RHEUMATISM – D. N. Golding
PROBLEMS IN CARDIOLOGY – C. F. P. Wharton
PROBLEMS IN GASTROENTEROLOGY – M. Lancaster-Smith and K. G. D. Williams
PROBLEMS IN GERIATRIC MEDICINE – A. Martin
PROBLEMS IN GYNAECOLOGY – E. P. W. Tatford
PROBLEMS IN OPHTHALMOLOGY – M. G. Glasspool
PROBLEMS IN OTOLARYNGOLOGY – P. Ratnesar
PROBLEMS IN PAEDIATRICS – J. Hood
PROBLEMS IN PERIPHERAL VASCULAR DISEASE – P. A. E. Savage
PROBLEMS IN RESPIRATORY MEDICINE – P. Forgacs
PROBLEMS IN SOCIAL CARE – J. Mogridge
SERIES INDEX VOLUME

Problems in Practice Series
Series Editors: J.Fry K.G.D.Williams M.Lancaster-Smith

Problems in Ophthalmology

Michael Glasspool
FRCS, DO

Consultant Ophthalmologist
Orpington Hospital, Kent

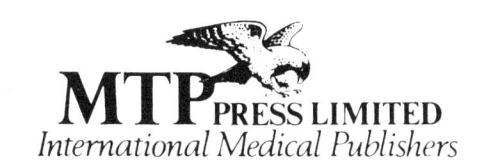

MTP PRESS LIMITED
International Medical Publishers

Published by
MTP Press Limited
Falcon House
Lancaster, England

Copyright © 1982 M. G. Glasspool

First published 1982

All rights reserved. No part of this publication
may be reproduced, stored in a retrieval
system, or transmitted in any form or by any
means, electronic, mechanical, photocopying,
recording or otherwise, without prior
permission from the publishers.

Glasspool, Michael
  Problems in ophthalmology.—(Problems in practice series)
  1. Ophthalmology
  I. Title   II. Series
  617.7   RE46

ISBN 0-85200-322-6

Phototypesetting by Swiftpages Limited, Liverpool and printed
by Redwood Burn Limited, Trowbridge.

Contents

	Series Foreword *J. P. Horder CBE*	7
1	**History**	9
2	**Examination**	17

Introduction – visual acuity – visual fields – colour vision – external examination – internal examination – opthalmoscopy

3 The red eye   31
Introduction – conjunctivitis – episcleritis – keratitis – iritis – acute glaucoma

4 The external eye   47
Introduction – lids – conjunctiva

5 The internal eye   53
Examination of the inner eye – alteration in pigment – toxoplasmosis – toxocara – opaque nerve fibres

6 Sudden loss of vision   59
Introduction – migraine – amaurosis fugax – renal artery occlusion – temporal arteritis – retinal vein occlusion – vitreous – retinal detachment

7 Slow loss of vision   67
Introduction – cataract – chronic glaucoma – macular degeneration

8 Trauma   99
Introduction – superficial injuries – lacerations – penetrating injuries – blunt injury – chemical injuries – radiation injuries

Problems in ophthalmology

9 Paediatric ophthalmology 113
Introduction – squint – watering eyes – ptosis – congenital glaucoma – retinoblastoma

10 The eye and systemic disease 119
Introduction – thyroid disease – the fundus – hypertension – diabetes – papilloedema – multiple sclerosis

11 Ocular pharmacology 129

Index 135

Series Foreword

This series of books is designed to help general practitioners. So are other books. What is unusual in this instance is their collective authorship; they are written by specialists working at district general hospitals. The writers derive their own experience from a range of cases less highly selected than those on which textbooks are traditionally based. They are also in a good position to pick out topics which they see creating difficulties for the practitioners of their district, whose personal capacities are familiar to them; and to concentrate on contexts where mistakes are most likely to occur. They are all well-accustomed to working in consultation.

All the authors write from hospital experience and from the viewpoint of their specialty. There are, therefore, matters important to family practice which should be sought not within this series, but elsewhere. Within the series much practical and useful advice is to be found with which the general practitioner can compare his existing performance and build in new ideas and improved techniques.

These books are attractively produced and I recommend them.

J. P. Horder CBE
President, The Royal College
of General Practitioners

1 History

A good history is as important in ophthalmology as in other branches of medicine. The patient should be allowed to tell his story and this, together with a few carefully chosen direct questions, can often give an accurate lead to the ultimate diagnosis. However, eye symptoms can be vague and when combined with the emotive nature of eye disease may result in misunderstanding.

Terminology

It must be remembered that some terms used by the layman may not mean the same to the doctor. The 'squinting eye' may only be screwed up and not imply any deviation, while 'double vision' may be used when the image is merely blurred.

Previous ocular disease

It is important to ask if there has been any previous ocular disease. A childhood squint may have resulted in a lazy eye and this defective vision can be overlooked until adult life, when investigation and treatment to try to improve the poor visual acuity would be useless.

Previous trauma may have caused changes in the ocular structures without significantly impairing the vision. Blunt injury to the eye commonly causes traumatic mydriasis with the affected pupil becoming permanently larger and less reactive than normal. This could be confused with a partial third cranial nerve palsy.

Cataracts produced by long-forgotten trauma may have caused opacities in part of the lens, which can be confused with changes of more recent onset.

General health

Many conditions of the eye are manifestations of systemic disease. Occasionally, the ocular complications develop only after the systemic ailment is well established. Such is the case with diabetes, in which retinal changes are not usually seen until the condition has been present for many years. Conversely, the ocular symptoms may precede more generalized symptoms.

Subconjunctival haemorrhage or sudden vitreous haemorrhage may be the presenting signs of hypertension, and iritis may appear before the low backache of the related ankylosing spondylitis.

All *drug therapy* should be recorded. Certain systemic drugs have well-known side-effects on the eye, such as corticosteroid-induced cataract, chloroquine retinopathy or ethambutol optic atrophy. These should present no problem providing the patient is adequately monitored. This usually involves regular attendance at an eye clinic for assessment by an ophthalmologist for as long as the drug is being administered. Any new ocular signs like the dry eye induced by practalol should be regarded with suspicion as complications may even appear after use of a drug for several years.

Family history   Certain eye conditions have a strong hereditary basis. Of these, *chronic glaucoma* is the most important, with the incidence being nearly five times greater in siblings and the children of affected patients. Recognition of these first degree relatives who are at risk together with suitable screening and early treatment can help reduce the morbidity of the condition.

A family history of *squint* should act as a warning not to ignore the possibility of further members of the same family being similarly affected.

Symptoms of Eye Disease

These fall into three main groups:

(1) vision
(2) sensation
(3) appearance.

Vision

Alteration of visual function provides the main clue for the solving of the majority of ocular problems.

If the patient does not volunteer the following facts, then direct questions should be put to him.

(1) *Does the problem affect one or both eyes?*

It is a common mistake for disturbances in the peripheral fields of vision to be noticed only in the temporal field and any nasal defect is ignored. So the visual loss in right-sided homony-

History

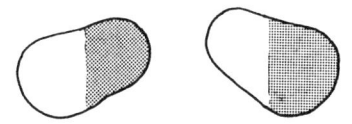

Diagram 1 Right-sided homonymous hemianopia. Left, nasal loss ignored (shaded area); right, temporal loss noticed (shaded area)

mous hemianopia is blamed on the right eye with the patient overlooking the nasal loss in the left eye (Diagram 1). Similarly, the visual disturbance with migraine may be thought by the patient to affect only one eye. He must, therefore, be asked if he has ever covered the affected side to check the fellow eye.

(2) *Was the visual loss sudden or gradual?*

Sudden visual loss occurring over seconds or minutes usually implies a vascular cause, while *gradual loss* over several days may be caused by retinal detachment. A much slower deterioration over months is usually the result of the development of cataract or macular changes.

Occasionally the complaint of sudden visual loss is made when the patient covers one eye and discovers the poor vision in the other eye which has been defective for many years, but which has passed unnoticed.

(3) *Is the visual loss complete or only partial?*

Cataract causes an overall mistiness in contrast to the dense central loss of vision found in macular disease, in which the peripheral vision is retained. Loss of the peripheral field of vision is associated with retinal detachment, chronic glaucoma and the visual field defects caused by intracranial lesions. (Diagram 2).

(4) *Is there any associated visual disturbance?*

Double vision when seen with two eyes is caused by a squint. Genuine double or even triple vision in one eye is a sign of early cataract formation.

Distortion of the central vision implies macular disease. Swelling of the retina in the macular area causes kinks in straight lines, micropsia (objects appearing smaller than normal) and occasionally disturbances of colour vision.

Flashing lights are common in migraine when a coloured zigzag-shaped line is seen in the centre of vision, which

Problems in ophthalmology

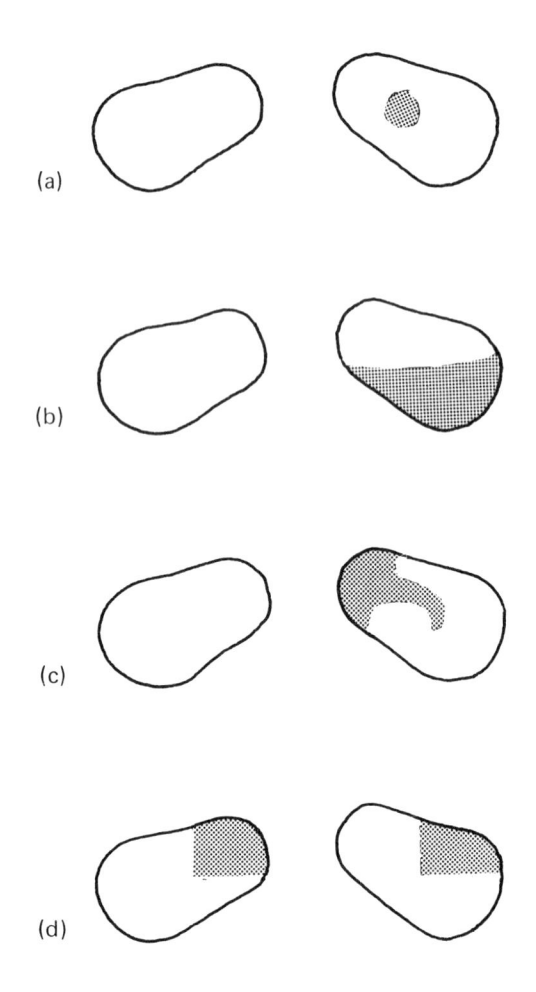

a, Macular loss. **b**, Upper half retinal detachment causing lower half loss. **c**, Arcuate defect of glaucoma. **d**, Right homonymous quadrantic field loss

Diagram 2

gradually expands to fill the peripheral field of vision. Arcs of light, sparks or flashes similar to lightning may herald a retinal detachment. These symptoms may be accompanied by the sudden appearance of *black floaters* or *cobwebs* as blood leaks into the vitreous. *Haloes* of rainbow-coloured lights may indicate subacute attacks of narrow angle glaucoma.

History

Sensation

Numerous epithets are used by patients to describe the sensations produced by ocular disease. These may be simplified to pain and discharge.

Pain

The localization of pain by the eye is very inaccurate. Three main types of pain exist: (1) superficial (foreign body), (2) deep (iritis) and (3) referred (headache).

Superficial pain

Superficial pain may be described as sharp, gritty or burning. It may be very severe, as anyone who has had a foreign body under the lid will know. The pain from a corneal lesion may be attributed to the upper lid, since the discomfort occurs when the lid is closed.

Superficial pain is relieved by local anaesthetic drops, which may be needed to overcome the spasm of the lids in order to perform an adequate examination of the eye.

Pain may occasionally be associated with irritation of the eyes, which is most commonly seen with allergic eye disease, notably hay fever and vernal conjunctivitis.

Superficial pain may be accompanied by dryness of the eyes, when the quantity of tears is reduced.

Deep pain

Deep pain is usually the result of an intraocular condition. Inflammation within the eye causes painful spasm of the pupil, which can be partially relieved by dilating the pupil with a mydriatic drug. Deep pain is described as being in or behind the eye and may vary from the dull ache of early iritis to the severe prostrating pain of acute glaucoma.

Referred pain

Referred pain due to intraocular conditions may radiate widely around the eye. Most commonly the pain is over the eyebrows, but it may also occur in the temporal or occipital regions. Very rarely does it radiate to or from the neck.

Headache is commonly attributed to eye disease, but in the majority of cases no ocular pathology can be found.

Eye strain due to a refractive error or to an imbalance of the action of the extraocular muscles accounts for a very small proportion of those patients complaining of headache. Such pain is usually related to use of the eyes, but it may be present on waking. It starts as a vague discomfort in or around the eyes, and increases in intensity to become a headache.

Photophobia or dislike of bright light may be present with any inflammatory condition of the conjunctiva or cornea. It is a characteristic early symptom in herpetic ulcers of the cornea, iritis and acute glaucoma.

Discharge

Tears
The commonest discharge from the eyes is excessive tears or epiphora. This may occur either due to overproduction of tears in response to irritation or more commonly to poor drainage.

Purulent
A sticky discharge which tends to glue the lashes together overnight is usually caused by staphylococcal infection. Rarely it is due to gonococci causing ophthalmia neonatorum with gross swelling of the lids, enlarged preauricular nodes and a purulent discharge.

Serous
A watery discharge suggests infection which is viral in origin. This is accompanied by painless enlargement of the local lymph nodes and the formation of follicles in the conjunctiva lining the lids.

Mucoid
Excess mucus from the conjunctival goblet cells tends to form as strings in the lower fornix, or to adhere to the cornea as fine filaments. This is typical of the dry eye of keratoconjunctivitis sicca.

Appearance

Alterations in the appearance of the eye may be due to changes either in the lids or the eyeball.

Lids

Normal appearance
The position of the normal upper lid just covers the upper 2–3 mm of cornea. The lower lid usually reaches the limbus (junction of the cornea and sclera).

Ptosis
Drooping or ptosis of the upper lid is usually apparent when the two eyes are compared. If there is no action of the levator palpebral muscle, the normal skin crease in the upper lid (the palpebral fold) is missing. If the ptosis is bilateral the abnormal position of the lid in relation to the cornea is noted.

Retraction
Retraction of the lids is obvious when a rim of sclera becomes visible between the lid and the cornea. Lid retraction is most commonly associated with thyroid eye disease. When the lower lid is involved proptosis of the eye is present due to the forward displacement of the globe by the increased orbital contents (thyroid disease, tumour or inflammation).

Swelling
Swelling of the lids may be localized, or may spread to

History

involve both lids and the cheek. The lids are easily distended and even minor localized infections can cause marked lid swelling, with complete closure of the eye. Oedema can even spread across the bridge of the nose to involve the opposite side of the face.

The eyeball

Position
Proptosis
Enophthalmos

Alteration of the position of the eyeball is most commonly seen when a squint is present. Proptosis, with forward displacement of the eye due to increased orbital contents, or enophthalmos, when the eye sinks into the orbit, are less common.

Conjunctival colour changes

Painless red discoloration may occur with subconjunctival haemorrhage; yellow staining of the conjunctival tissues may be part of more generalized changes caused by jaundice.

Scleral colour changes

Changes in the colour of the sclera may be due to thinning of the scleral layers so that the underlying choroid becomes visible. Slate-grey discoloration may occur as an ageing change when it appears on the medial and lateral sides, or more extensively when associated with rheumatoid arthritis.

2 Examination

Introduction – Visual acuity – Visual fields – Colour vision – External examination – Internal examination – Ophthalmoscopy

Introduction

The combination of insufficient time and inadequate equipment often means that examination of the eyes is perfunctory. The scant information gained does little to further the possible diagnosis and even less for the doctor's feeling of a job well done.

However, it is possible, in a short time, with a minimum of suitable equipment and a modicum of knowledge, to be able to decide the management of the majority of common eye conditions.

Equipment   Assuming that there is adequate general illumination in the room, the following items are necessary:

(1) Snellen chart
(2) Ophthalmoscope
(3) Magnifying glass
(4) Fluorescein strips, tropicamide and oxybuprocaine (Benoxinate) drops.

Visual acuity

Snellen chart   Assessment of the visual acuity can be performed with the traditional 6 metre Snellen chart if there is room for the patient to be seated at the correct distance (6 metres from the chart).

Problems in ophthalmology

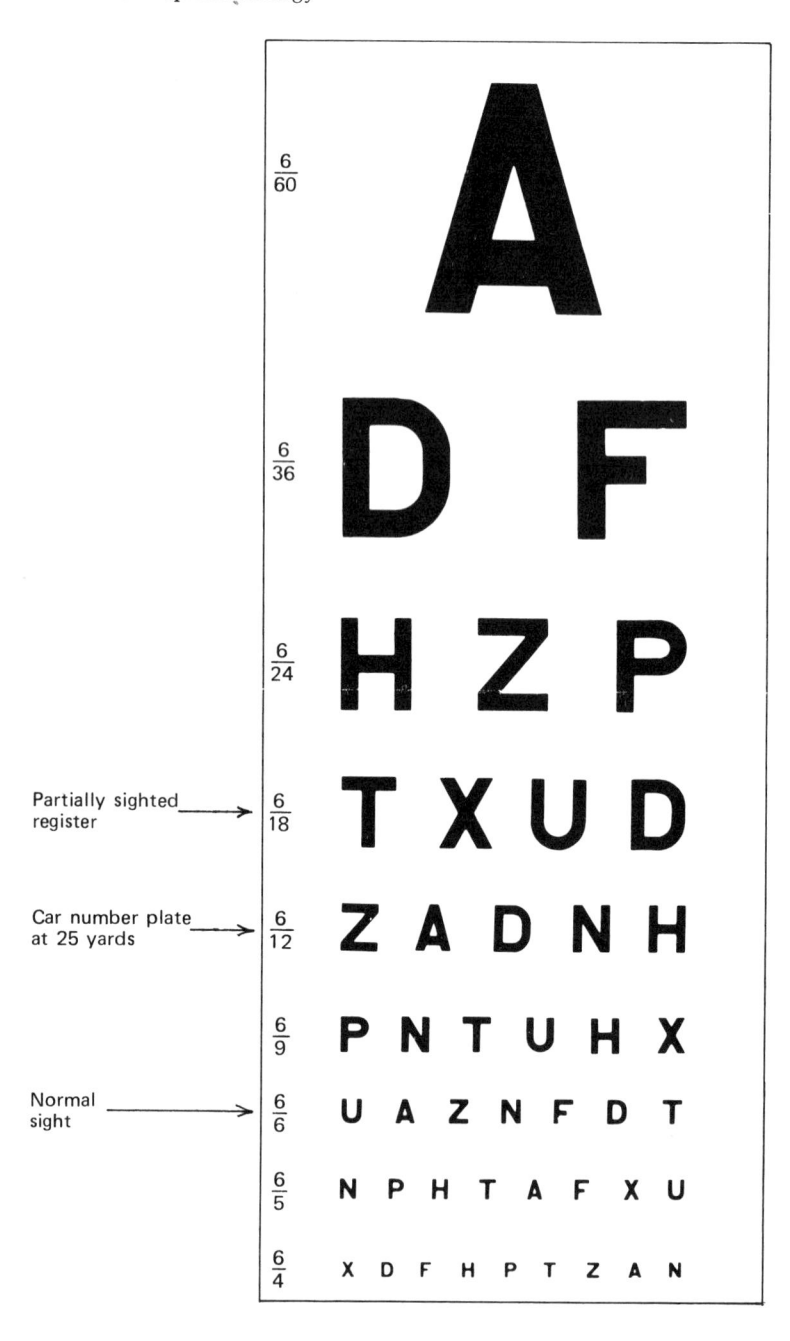

	$\frac{6}{60}$ **A**
	$\frac{6}{36}$ **D F**
	$\frac{6}{24}$ **H Z P**
Partially sighted register →	$\frac{6}{18}$ **T X U D**
Car number plate at 25 yards →	$\frac{6}{12}$ **Z A D N H**
	$\frac{6}{9}$ **P N T U H X**
Normal sight →	$\frac{6}{6}$ **U A Z N F D T**
	$\frac{6}{5}$ **N P H T A F X U**
	$\frac{6}{4}$ **X D F H P T Z A N**

A Snellen chart, which must be 6 metres from the patient (reproduced 35% of full size)

Diagram 1

Examination

Method

Alternatively, the patient can view the chart reflected in a mirror placed at 3 metres, so that the distance from chart to mirror to patient totals 6 metres. A convenient method is using a reduced Snellen chart on which the letters are proportionately smaller so that the chart can be placed 3 metres away.

If he or she uses glasses, the patient should wear his or her distance correction. Some patients will mistakenly wear their reading glasses on the grounds that they are reading letters, regardless of the distance from the chart, or will remove their glasses to facilitate the examination by the doctor.

One eye is covered, preferably using a piece of card, as it is quite possible to peep between the fingers if the hand is used. The patient is then asked to read from the top to the lowest line. Patients often stop one or even two lines short of their best; suitable encouragement therefore is necessary. The fellow eye is then tested.

Results

The results are recorded from 6/60 – the top letter to 6/6 – normal (Diagram 1).

The numerator 6 refers to the distance from the patient to the chart and the denominator to the line which he can see. So 6/18 means that from 6 metres away he or she can see the line which the normal person can read at 18 metres. In practice, the standard 6/6 can usually be exceeded by the majority of patients who are able to read 6/5 or even 6/4.

In the USA the distances are measured in feet so that 6/6 is equivalent to 20/20, while in Continental Europe a decimal notation is used (Table 2.1).

Table 2.1 Visual acuity assessment measurement systems

Snellen (metres)	USA (feet)	Europe (decimal)
6/6	20/20	1.0
6/9	20/30	0.7
6/12	20/40	0.5
6/18	20/60	0.3
6/24	20/80	0.25
6/60	20/200	0.1

Pinhole test

When the visual acuity is below normal, the test should be repeated with the patient looking through a 1 mm or 2 mm hole in a piece of card. This acts by allowing only a very narrow pencil of rays to enter the eye. If the vision improves, then the patient should be referred for a test for glasses, but if there is no improvement, further examination is necessary.

Problems in ophthalmology

N.5

Such very small print as this is used only for special cases, for example, the small advertisements and financial columns in some magazines, for indexes and references, and pocket-sized bibles and prayerbooks.

ewers—save—seam—crease

N.6

This type size, the smallest in general use, is used in some newspapers for the classified advertisements, in telephone directories and timetables, and other such lists and reference books.

museum—cone—nave—sun

N.8

Most of the daily newspapers use this as the average size of print for their news columns. The letters are sometimes larger than this, but rarely are they smaller.

crown—serve—seen—newer

N.10

Magazines, novels and textbooks are usually set in characters of about this size, as are printed instructions.

ream—ear—venom—ruse

N.12

Books which are printed on very large pages, with many words on each line, often use a type similar to this one.

mane—sue—smear—sores

N.14

Titles of book and headings to paragraphs in newspapers are often set in type of this size, but usually in CAPITAL LETTERS.

mere—crane—oar—summer

N.18

BOLD headlines and children's books.

rose—one—scour—never

N.24

ADVERTISEMENTS, display.

Diagram 2 Near-vision test type. Letter size ranges from N.5 to N.24

Examination

When the patient is unable to read the top letter, he should attempt to count the fingers of the examiner's hand held at 1 metre or 50 cm. This is recorded as counting fingers (C.F.). If the patient is unable to do this, the examiner should move his whole hand in front of the eye to record hand movements (H.M.). Failing this, a light is shone onto the eye for perception of light (P.L.). The direction of the light may be varied to stimulate the different areas of the retina.

Near vision   To measure near vision a test type should be held at 30 cm in a good light (Diagram 2). The test uses Times Roman print in sizes from 5 to 48 point. The near acuity is recorded by the prefix letter N (near) to give N.5–N.48.

Wearing reading glasses, if they are used, the patient should be able to see the smallest letters – N.5. If the distance vision is below normal the near vision is usually reduced.

A rough guide can be obtained by dividing the distance vision by three. Accordingly, with 6/24 distance vision the patient should be able to read N.8 and seeing 6/18 can manage N.6.

Visual fields

The presence of a field defect may be noticed by the patient and can be a presenting symptom. This is found with the loss of vision in retinal detachment or vascular occlusions of the retina. More often, the patient is unaware of the loss of vision, but may complain merely of difficulty in seeing either for distance or near.

Difficulty with reading   A right-sided homonymous hemianopia may cause reading problems as the eyes are unable to scan along the line of words due to the blind area on the right side. Problems are also experienced with a left-sided homonymous field defect when it becomes difficult to find the beginning of the next line of print.

Difficulty with distance vision   An indication of similar field defects may be given when the visual acuity is tested. The patient reads only one side of the Snellen chart and ignores those letters on the same side as the loss of vision.

Confrontation method   Accurate charting of central and peripheral fields of vision is only possible with the equipment that is found in eye clinics. However, the confrontation method can be used as a rough guide to possible field defects.

The doctor and patient sit facing each other about 1 metre apart (**Figure 2.1**, p. 33). With the patient covering his right eye and the doctor his left, the peripheral visual field of the doctor can then be compared with that of the patient. The uncovered eye of the patient can be watched to make certain that he does not move the eye. He should be asked to say when he sees movement of the doctor's fingers. The opposite eye is then covered and the test repeated. This method can be used to detect only large areas of loss of the field of vision, which extend to the extreme periphery. Loss in the central field can be detected using an old-fashioned hatpin, but the test is inaccurate and requires considerable concentration by the patient.

In general, if any field defect is elicited by the confrontation method the patient should be referred for more detailed examination.

Colour vision

Tests for colour discrimination are numerous, but the Ishihara Isochromatic plates are amongst the simplest to use. A set of plates is viewed by the patient under daylight conditions. Each plate consists of a series of small dots of differing colours arranged so that the normal eye can see the outline of a number amongst the dots. The test will detect those patients with the commoner red/green colour deficiency that is found with retrobulbar neuritis and toxic amblyopia.

External examination

Skin Skin changes may suggest rosacea, or molluscum contagiosum, either of which may be the underlying cause of a chronically irritable eye.

Facial symmetry External examination of the eyes should include the whole face. The symmetry of the face can be gauged by drawing an imaginary vertical line down the centre of the nose. It is then easier to judge the relative positions of each eye, cheek and angle of the mouth. Sometimes an apparent squint may be due to a small degree of facial asymmetry and not to any true ocular deviation. Broadening of the bridge of the nose associated with epicanthic folds can also cause a pseudosquint. Flattening of the cheek bone may occur with a fracture of the malar bones.

Muscle weakness Weakness of the facial nerve may show by loss of the labial fold, the skin crease running from the nose to the angle of the mouth. When the orbicularis oculi muscle is involved, the patient may be unable to close the lids completely, resulting in lagophthalmos.

Examination

Position of eyeballs

The position of the eyeballs can be judged by holding a straight edge horizontally in line with first the lower and then the upper lids.

Vertical displacement of the eyeball may be the result of trauma, tumour or inflammation, or may be merely due to congenital asymmetry. The cause of the displacement may be helped by referring to old photographs to ascertain its duration.

Lids' normal position

The normal position of the lower lid is against the limbus (the junction of cornea and sclera) while the upper lid usually overlaps the cornea by 1–2 mm.

Ptosis

Ptosis or drooping of the upper lid is caused by weakness of the levator muscle. It may be accompanied by complete loss of the skin crease over the eye (palpebral fold) and occasionally by the overaction of the frontalis muscle so that the eyebrow is raised.

Lid retraction

Retraction of the upper and lower lids is marked by the appearance of a rim of sclera visible between the limbus and the lid margin. When the upper lid is retracted, thyrotoxicosis is the commonest cause. Retraction of the lower lid implies a forward displacement of the eyeball (proptosis or exophthalmos).

Ocular movements

Examination of the ocular movements for a possible squint, unless it is very obvious, usually produces a complete mental block in many doctors. This is unnecessary if a set pattern of examination is carried out and a few basic anatomical facts are remembered.

The squinting eye may be obvious, with the cornea directed towards the nose and more sclera visible laterally than normal in the convergent squint. The reverse findings occur for the divergent eye.

Method of cover test

To detect a small squint the cover test is necessary. The patient is asked to look at the ophthalmoscope light. The right eye is then covered while the left is watched for any movement.

Manifest squint

If the left eye moves inwards a manifest left *divergent* squint is present (Diagram 3a), if the movement is outwards a *convergent* squint exists (Diagram 3b).

If there is no movement the test is repeated covering the left eye and watching for movement in the right eye.

Latent squint

A latent squint is detected by the same test. However, observation is kept on the covered eye to see if there is any movement when it is uncovered. A latent convergent or divergent squint will be present if the eye moves to a central position when it is uncovered.

Paralytic squint

Knowing the relevant anatomical details, recalled below, and by following the movement of the ophthalmoscope light it is

Problems in ophthalmology

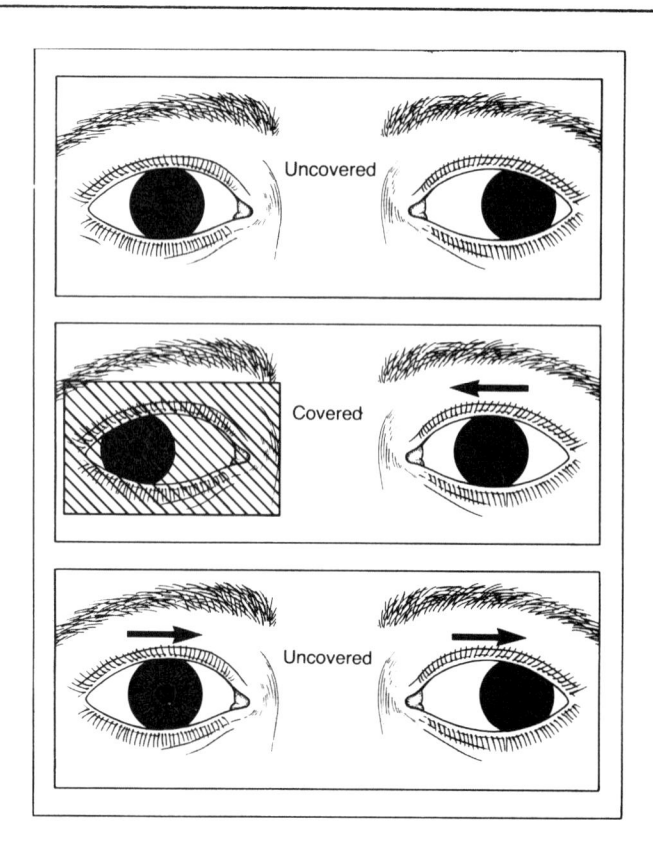

Diagram 3a Left divergent squint. Movements of the eyes with the cover test are shown

possible to localize the affected cranial nerve in a paralytic squint.

The extraocular muscles are supplied by the third, fourth and sixth cranial nerves.

(1) The sixth cranial nerve supplies the lateral rectus muscle which abducts the eye.

(2) The fourth cranial nerve supplies the superior oblique muscle which moves the eye downwards and inwards.

(3) The third cranial nerve supplies the remaining muscles which move the eye in all other directions. It also supplies the levator muscle of the upper lid and the constrictor fibres of the iris muscle.

Examination

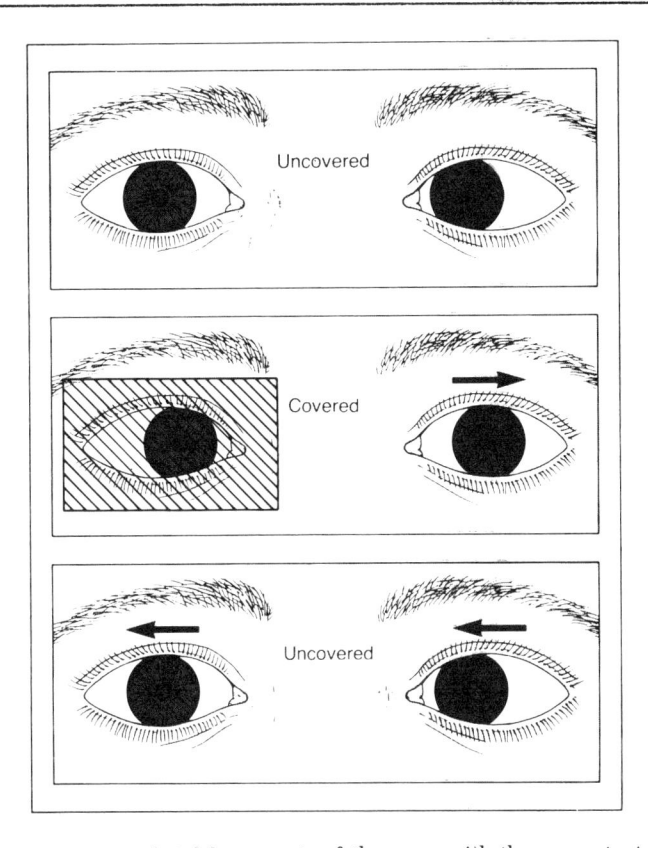

Left convergent squint. Movements of the eyes with the cover test are shown

Diagram 3b

Pupil reactions

Direct reaction
Consensual reaction

Near reflex

Convergence

The normal pupil reactions can be tested using the light of the ophthalmoscope. The patient is instructed to look at the distance test chart and the light is shone directly in front of the eye. The direct pupillary reaction consists of a brisk maintained constriction of the pupil. The consensual reaction is seen in the opposite eye at the same time as the direct reaction.

The near reflex is elicited by asking the patient to look into the distance and then to look at the tip of a pen held 10–15 cm away. The pupillary constriction is less marked than the response to light.

The ability to converge on a near object is assessed by the ease with which the patient can keep both eyes fixed on an object as it is gradually brought closer to the eyes. Convergence

Problems in ophthalmology

Magnifying glass   to within 10 cm can normally be achieved before the patient sees double.

Closer examination of the lids and eyeball is helped by using a magnifying lens and the light of the ophthalmoscope. In order to obtain adequate magnification, the focal length and, therefore, the working distance must be very short. Accordingly it is necessary not only to hold the lens near the eye, but to get as near to the lens as possible in order to get a large field of vision.

Lids

The lids should be examined for any displacement of the lashes or punctum. The lower lid must be pulled down while the patient looks up to see the conjunctival lining and the lower fornix.

Eversion of lid

The upper lid must be everted in order not to miss small retained foreign bodies. To do this the lashes are held firmly while counterpressure is applied to the upper border of the tarsal plate 1 cm from the lid margin. At the same time the lashes are lifted gently forwards and upwards (**Figure 2.2**, p. 33). The manoeuvre is made easier if the patient is told to keep looking down.

Cornea

The normal cornea is bright and clear. The bright-light reflex is due partly to the tear film and in part to the optical clarity of the corneal tissues. The tear strip along the lower lid margin is obviously enlarged when there is excessive tearing (epiphora), and is diminished or absent if the tear secretion is defective.

The optical clarity of the cornea is due to a number of factors. Externally, intact epithelium covers the avascular corneal stroma which is prevented from becoming waterlogged by a healthy endothelium lining the inside of the cornea.

Epithelium

Damage to the epithelium causes considerable pain and examination may only be possible after use of a weak anaesthetic (oxybuprocaine (Minims Benoxinate Hydrochloride)). Large ulcers or abrasions are readily visible with good illumination and a magnifying lens, but smaller lesions may be difficult to see. The instillation of fluorescein dye will delineate any abrasion and is more readily visible if lit with a blue light. It is unwise to use fluorescein drops which tend to stain not only the eye but also the face as well. The most convenient method is using a sterile impregnated strip of paper (Fluoret), which is placed inside the lower lid. The normal tear secretion is sufficient to wet the paper and the dye is distributed over the eye by a few blinks.

Stroma

There are numerous causes for the opacities that may be seen in the stroma. Arcus senilis may occur as an ageing change

Examination

in the peripheral cornea, while central scarring is common after herpetic keratitis.

Many stromal lesions are more easily seen when the pupil is dilated, so that the affected cornea is viewed with the black pupil as a background.

Endothelium Changes in the endothelium are not usually visible even with a magnifying lens. Keratic precipitates (K.P.) may be seen in iritis if the aggregations of white cells are large.

Internal examination

Anterior chamber The depth of the anterior chamber must be assessed before the pupil is dilated. If the patient wears hypermetropic spectacles
Long sight with magnifying or plus lenses, the eye is usually shorter than normal and the anterior chamber is liable to be shallow.

Short sight For the myopic patient the reverse occurs, with the elongated eye being associated with a deep anterior chamber.

Method Using direct illumination from the ophthalmoscope it is possible to see in the normal eye the iris lying well away from the cornea forming an angle of 45°. When the anterior chamber is shallow the iris appears convex and the separation of the iris and cornea seems no greater in the centre of the anterior chamber than in the periphery. The iris may even seem to be lining the inside of the cornea.

Lens Examination of the lens by direct illumination should reveal an apparently black area in the pupil. If there are any opacities these may appear as whitish flecks in the black pupil. With increasing age the black appearance may be tinged with yellow or brown as the lens becomes hard. Using an ophthalmoscope it becomes possible to see further details in the lens as the examination of the fundus is performed.

Ophthalmoscopy

There is a wide choice of ophthalmoscopes ranging from the more complex specialist models to the simple pocket versions.

The Keeler Practitioner or Pocket models both may be combined with an otoscope as diagnostic sets. They have the advantage of providing a satisfactory range of lenses together with a macular beam, which allows examination of the macula through an undilated pupil.

Regardless of which ophthalmoscope is chosen, great care must be taken with its maintenance if the best possible view of the eye is to be obtained. The instrument must be kept free of dust and the batteries changed as soon as there is any sign of their failing. In addition the bulb should be examined periodically to exclude blackening of the glass, which also reduces the level of illumination.

Dilating the pupils is necessary if a full examination of the peripheral retina is required. If, however, only the disc and immediate surrounding retina needs to be viewed, this can be achieved without dilation.

Tropicamide 0.5%–1% drops (Mydriacyl) produce adequate dilation in 10 minutes without severely affecting accommodation and wear off in 6 hours. Cyclopentolate 0.5% or 1% drops (Mydrilate) last longer and reduce accommodation unpleasantly.

The use of any stronger mydriatic drops should be avoided.

The risk of producing acute glaucoma is inadequate reason for not dilating the pupils.

Method

The method of examination is as follows.

(1) Set the ophthalmoscope at 0. If the examiner is myopic he should remove his own glasses and dial an equivalent strength of black or minus lens. If he is longsighted he must use the appropriate red or plus lens. To attempt ophthalmoscopy while wearing glasses prevents the examiner from holding the ophthalmoscope close enough to his own eye.

(2) Examine the patient's right eye with the ophthalmoscope held in the right hand. The left hand should be placed on the patient's head with the thumb retracting the upper lid. To examine the patient's left eye, learn to look with the left eye holding the ophthalmoscope with the left hand and steadying the patient's head with the right hand.

(3) With the patient looking straight ahead when viewed from 30 cm, the red reflex from the fundus is visible. Any opacities in the cornea, lens or vitreous will be silhouetted against the red reflex.

(4) Approach the patient slightly from the temporal side rather than from straight ahead, and aim at the centre of the head. This should bring the disc into view. If not, find a blood vessel and follow it back to the disc. The closer the examiner is to the patient, the larger will be the area of retina that is seen, and the easier it will be to see the major landmarks of the fundus.

Examination

(5) If the patient is shortsighted black or minus lenses will be needed to produce a sharp view of the fundus. In the longsighted patient it is possible for the examiner to accommodate and see the fundus details clearly.

(6) Follow the main blood vessels from the disc to the upper and lower nasal and temporal quadrants. It will be helpful to ask the patient to look in the direction of the quadrant which is being examined, so that the peripheral retina can be seen without unnecessary contortions by the examiner.

(7) The macula is seen when the patient is asked to look at the ophthalmoscope light. With the undilated pupil it is necessary to use a macular beam to prevent the intense pupillary constriction. When the pupil is dilated a broader beam can be used. The avascular macular area is about the same size as the disc. In the centre is the fovea which appears as a minute shining reflection of the ophthalmoscope light.

Intraocular pressure

A simple assessment of the intraocular pressure is possible using the digital method. The eye is palpated by the index fingers of each hand while the other fingers steady the hands by resting on the forehead (**Figure 2.3**, p. 33). This method is useful when the pressure in one eye is markedly raised, as in cases of acute glaucoma. Then the stony-hard eye can easily be compared with the normal eye.

Small rises in pressure cannot be detected using this method.

Conclusions

A routine should be observed for all patients who present with an ocular complaint. The time taken can be short since the eye is readily accessible and there is no delay caused by the patient undressing.

(1) Visual acuity:
 (a) Distance
 (b) Near
(2) Visual fields – if indicated by the history
(3) External examination
(4) Ophthalmoscopy.

3 The red eye

Introduction – Conjunctivitis – Episcleritis – Keratitis – Iritis – Acute glaucoma

Introduction

Redness of the eye with variable discomfort or pain is one of the commonest presentations of ocular problems. The importance of making the correct diagnosis at the first examination cannot be overemphasized. Incorrect diagnosis may result in potentially dangerous treatment, which can lead to permanent loss of sight.

Causes   There are five main groups into which the painful red eye can be divided:

(1) Conjunctivitis
(2) Episcleritis
(3) Keratitis
(4) Iritis
(5) Acute glaucoma.

Conjunctivitis

The term 'conjunctivitis' is most often applied to those cases with an infective origin, but it must be remembered that there are many other causes of 'inflammation of the conjunctiva'.

Causes   Bacteria and viruses are infective causes, while drugs, cosmetics, pollens and dust may produce an allergic reaction.

Symptoms   Each tends to present variations of the following main symptoms: (1) redness, (2) discharge and (3) pain.

Redness   Dilation of the conjunctival vessels is most easily seen on

Problems in ophthalmology

the sclera. Individual conjunctival vessels can be identified showing that it is the superficial tissues that are affected (**Figure 3.1**, p. 34). The whole of the conjunctival covering of the sclera may be reddened and the lining of the lids also becomes involved.

Conjunctivitis is usually a bilateral condition and redness of one eye is more likely to be due to inflammation of the cornea or iris, or to acute glaucoma.

Discharge
: Discharge may be purulent, serous or mucous, depending on the cause.

Pain
: Pain tends to be a grittiness rather than a pain and is made worse by movement of the eyes or lids. When the inflammation is allergic in origin, there may be accompanying irritation.

Bacterial infection
: Bacterial infection usually produces sticky red eyes. The lids are swollen and the lashes are stuck together, making it difficult to open the eyes on waking.

The redness tends to be generalized and the inside of the lids has a velvet-red appearance.

Occasionally, the infection may spread to the cornea to produce small white dots just within the limbus (marginal keratitis). These may coalesce to produce larger grey ulcers.

Causes
: The bacteria most commonly responsible are *Staphylococcus aureus* with the pneumococcus less common.

Treatment
: Ideally, local antibiotic treatment should not be started without first taking a conjunctival culture. In practice, it is rarely necessary. If there is doubt and the clinical signs are atypical, or because of medical legal reasons, the swab should be transferred to a blood agar plate.

Chloramphenicol is the drug of choice with the widest range of bacterial sensitivities. It should be given hourly in drops by day, with ointment at night. After the first 48 hours the drops may be reduced to four times each day. Treatment should continue for 5–7 days. Padding of the eyes should be avoided because the warmth behind the closed lids forms ideal conditions for bacterial multiplication. The use of ointment during the day is to be avoided as it causes unnecessary blurring of vision.

Gentacin, while more expensive, has a similar antibacterial range of activities and is also effective against *Pseudomonas* infection.

Viral infection
: Viral infection causes a diffusely red eye with gritty discomfort and a watery discharge. The inside of the lids show follicle formation caused by the aggregation of lymphocytes. The follicles appear as minute, clear, jelly-like blobs lining partic-

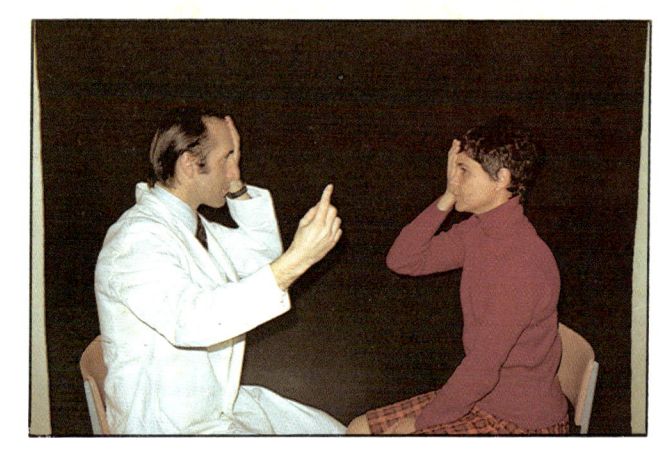

Figure 2.1

Confrontation test. A simple test for peripheral field loss requiring no equipment

Figure 2.2

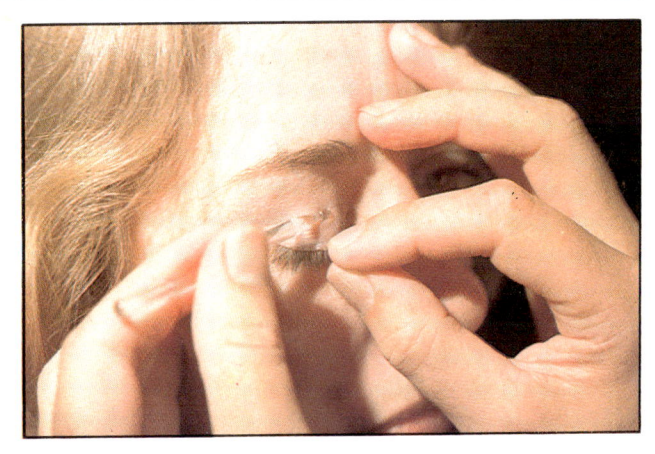

Eversion of the upper lid. Counterpressure is applied on the lid while the lashes are pulled upwards

Figure 2.3

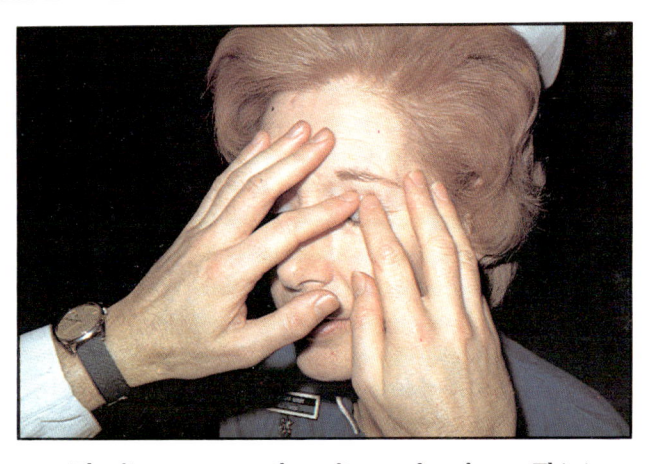

Digital tonometry. The fingers assess the softness of each eye. This is an inaccurate method but is useful for acute glaucoma

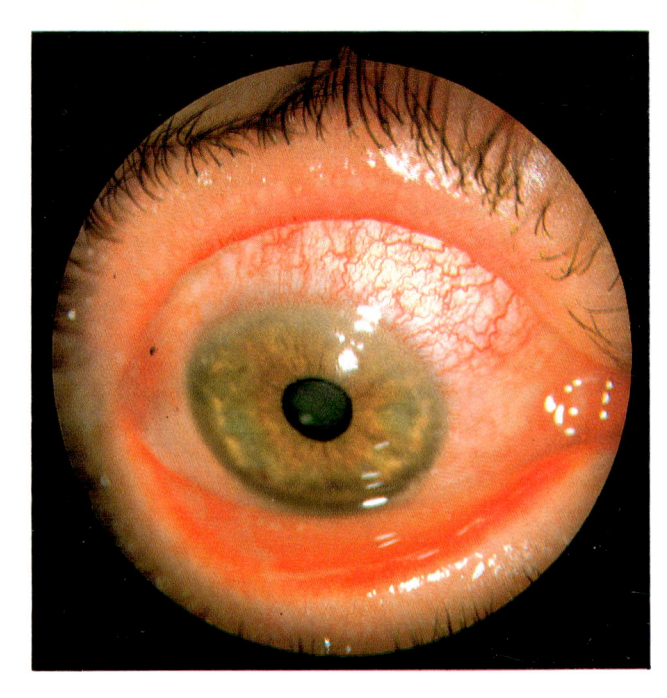

Figure 3.1 Conjunctivitis: injection of superficial conjunctival vessels

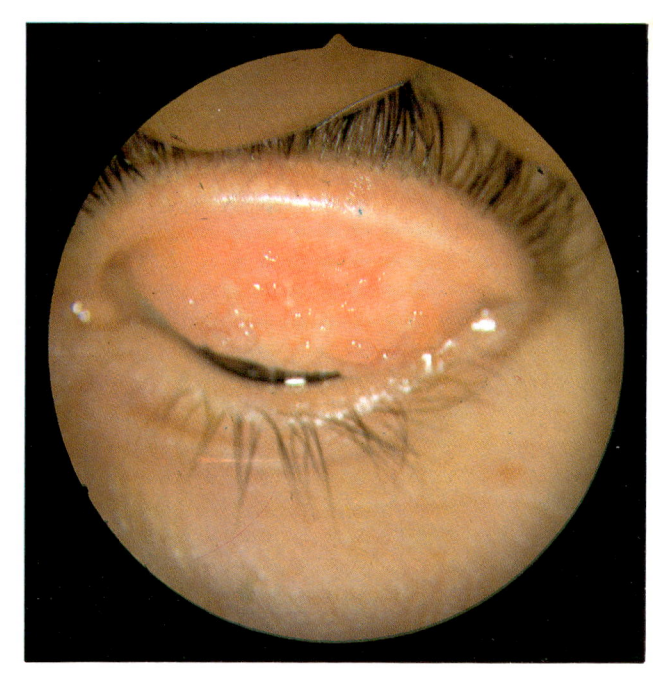

Figure 3.2 Vernal conjunctivitis: 'cobblestone' appearance from papillary overgrowth

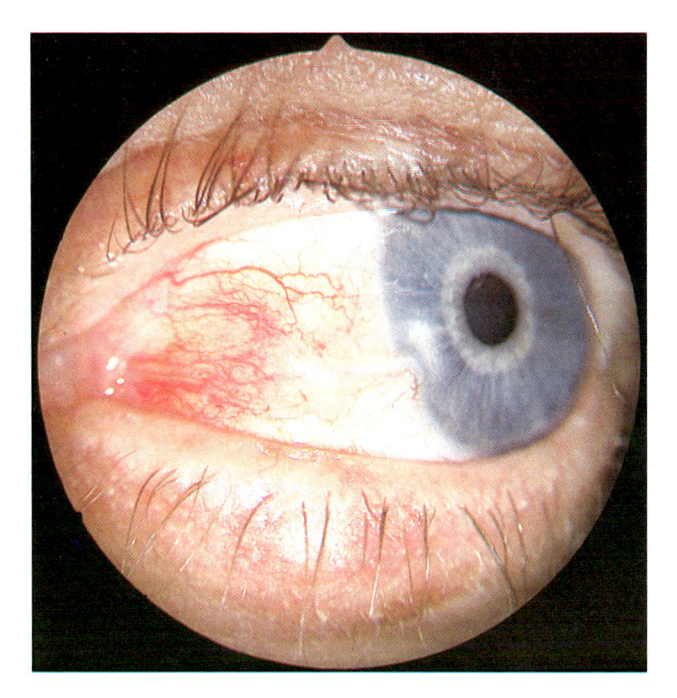

Figure 3.3 Episcleritis: segmental redness with a nodule adjacent to the cornea

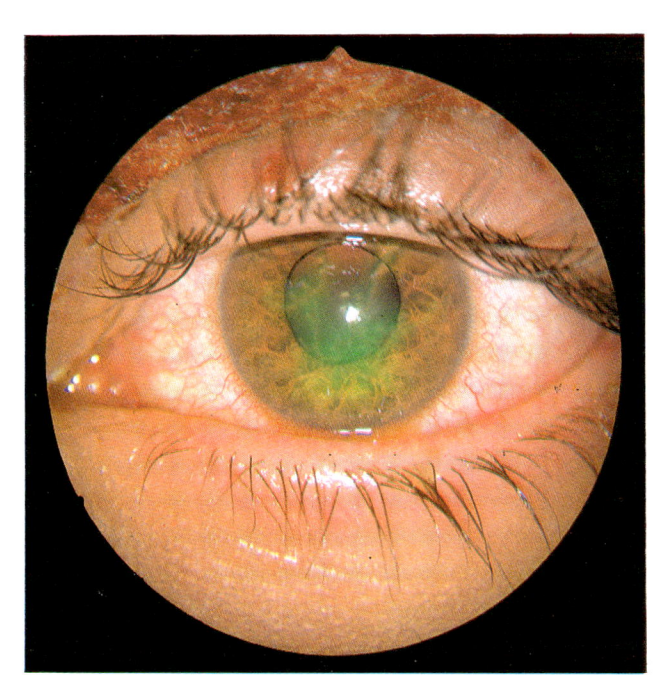

Figure 3.4 Dendritic ulcer: branching pattern of the ulcer which stains with fluorescein dye

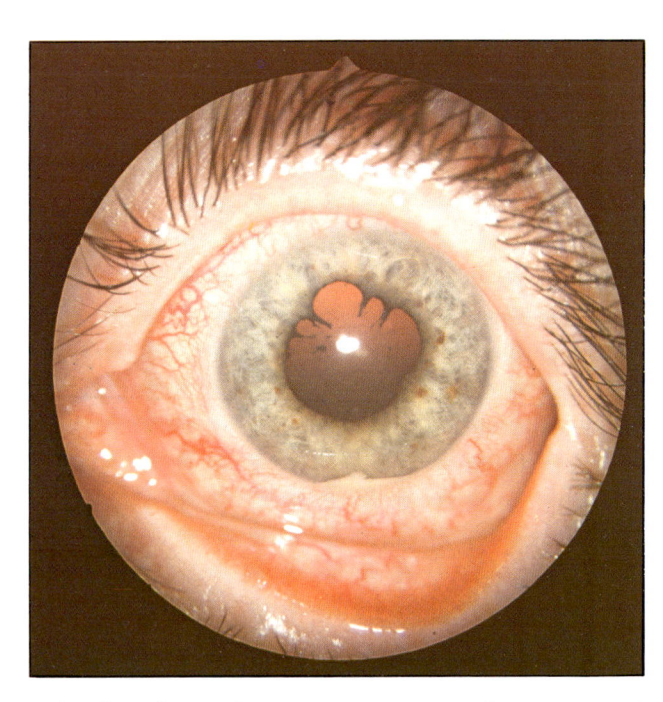

Figure 3.5 Uveitis: generalized redness, keratic precipitates, hypopyon and posterior synechiae are all hallmarks of anterior uveitis

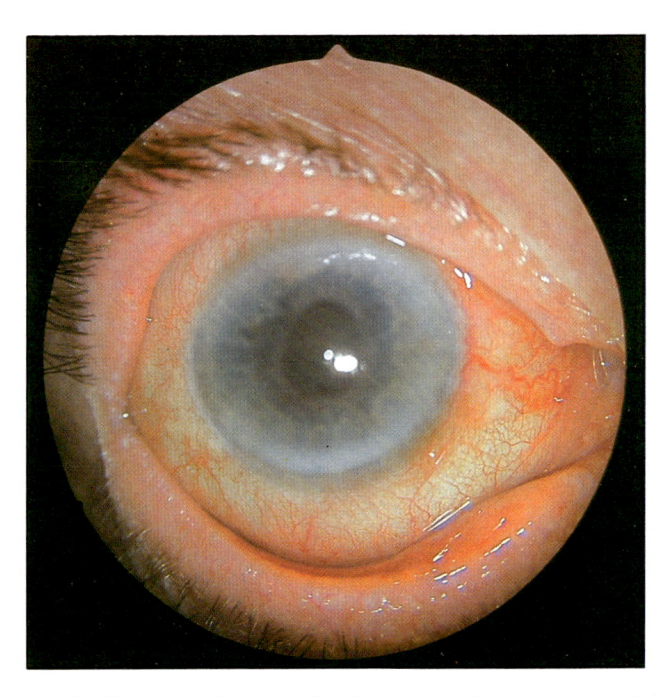

Figure 3.6 Acute narrow angle glaucoma: the typical red eye with a hazy cornea and a fixed and vertically oval pupil

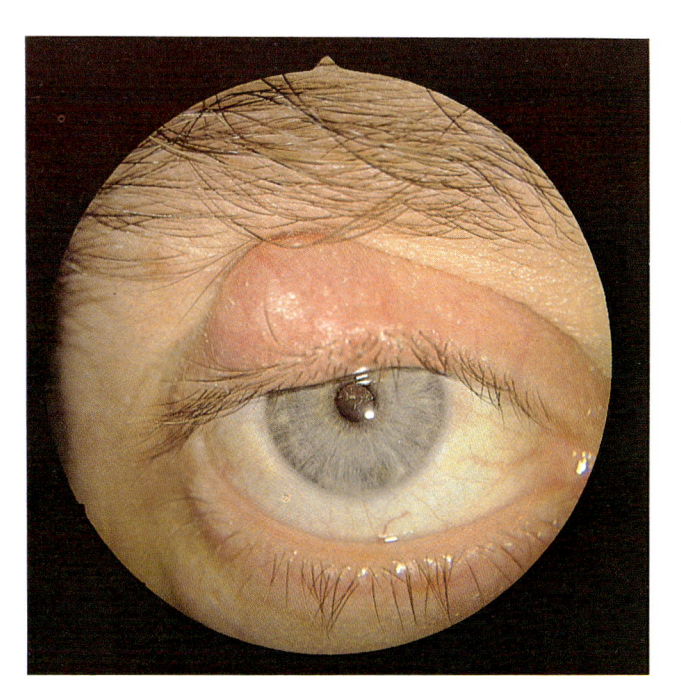

Figure 4.1 Chalazion: swelling of the cyst is behind the lid margin

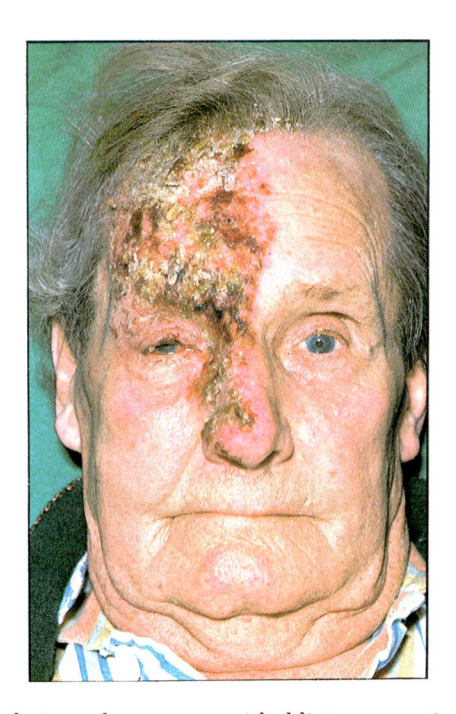

Figure 4.2 Herpes zoster ophthalmicus: late stage with blisters crusting over. Lesions on the tip of the nose with ocular involvement

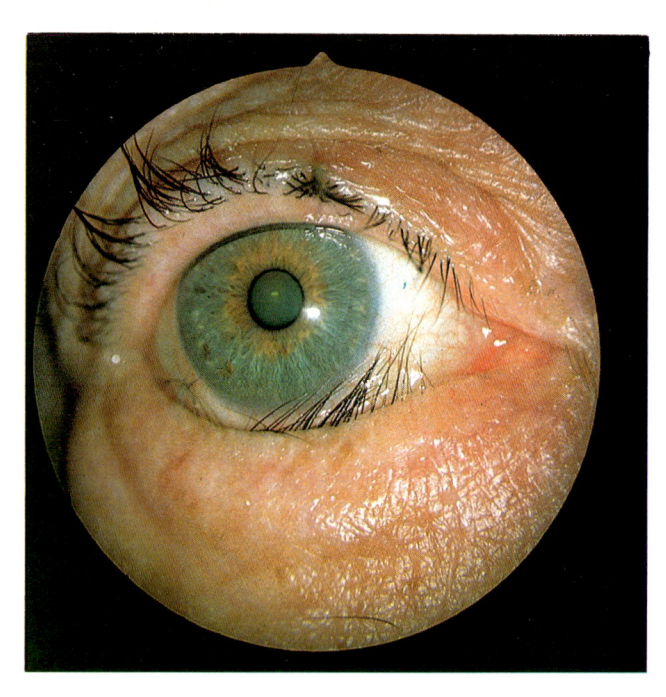

Figure 4.3 Entropion: lower lid is turned inwards so that the lashes are rubbing on the cornea

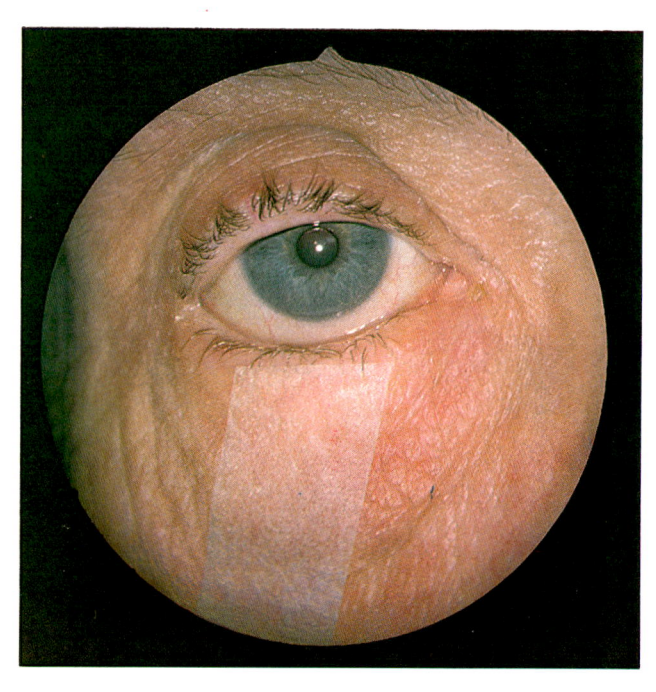

Figure 4.4 Entropion: emergency treatment with strapping to evert the lid

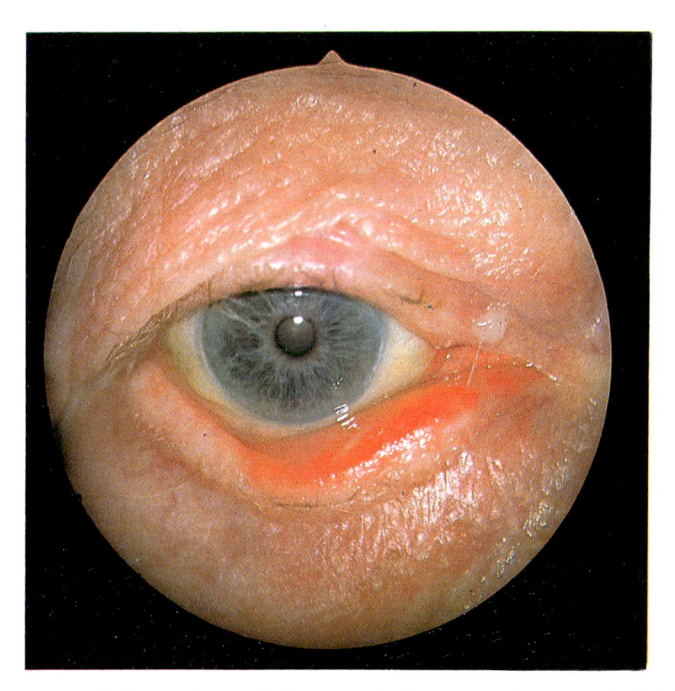

Ectropion: medial two thirds of the lower lid are turned outwards. Thickening of inner surface tends to increase the deformity

Figure 4.5

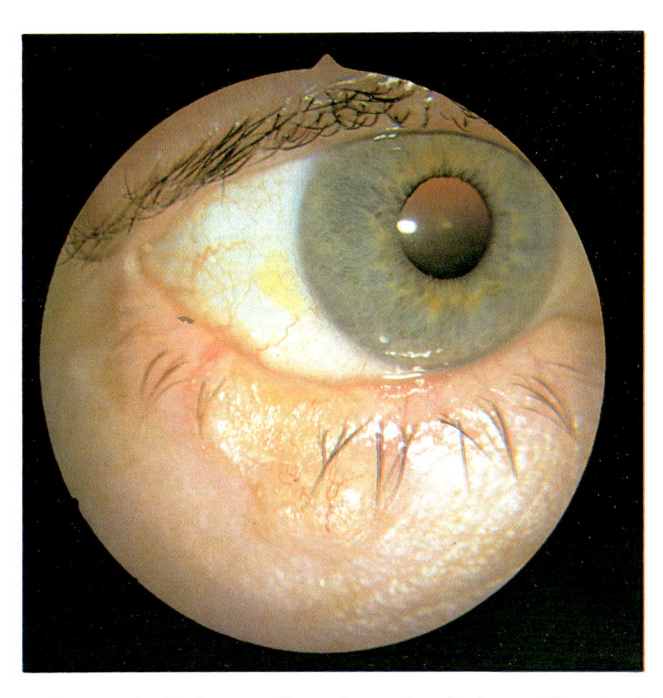

Basal cell carcinoma: typical spreading ulcerating lesion with raised edges, involving margin of lid

Figure 4.6

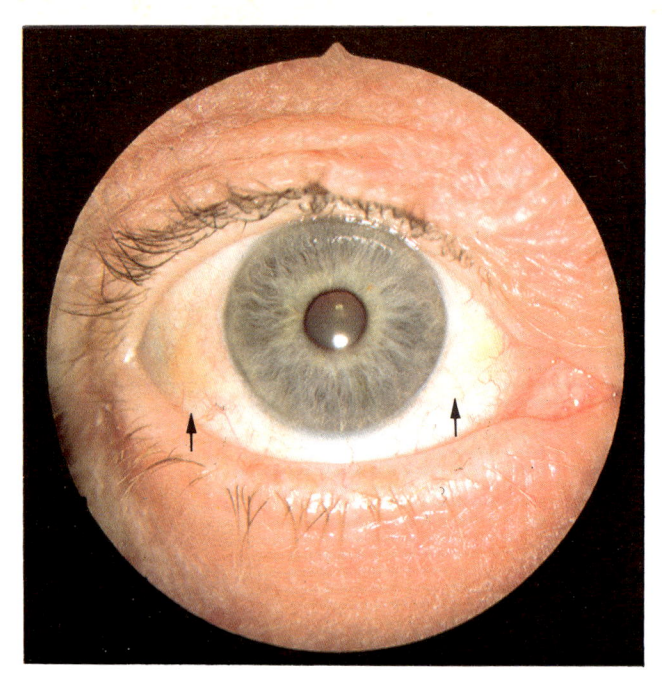

Figure 4.7 Pinguecula: yellowish degenerative lesions on the exposed sclera adjacent to the limbus

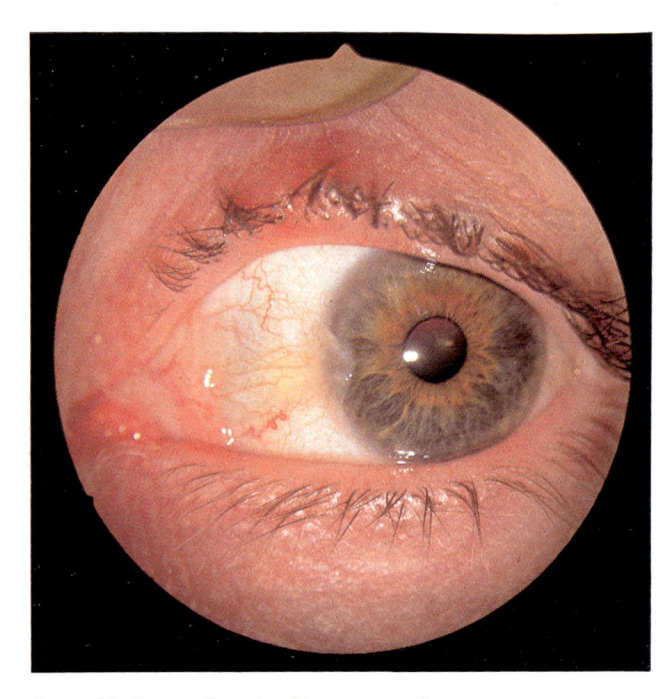

Figure 4.8 Pterygium: a 'wing-like' growth extending across the cornea

The red eye

ularly the lower lid, but not affecting the conjunctiva over the sclera.

Causes — The adenoviruses, especially numbers 3 and 8, herpes simplex and TRIC agents (TR for trachoma, IC for inclusion conjunctivitis) are the most commonly met.

Adenovirus — Adenovirus infection may be associated with an upper respiratory tract infection, pyrexia and enlarged preauricular glands. In addition to the follicular conjunctivitis the cornea may have multiple small whitish opacities.

Treatment with local antibiotic drops for any secondary infection is usually all that is required. The condition is self-limiting over several weeks. If there are corneal changes the patient should be referred for treatment. As the condition is so contagious, great care should be taken after any examination.

Herpes simplex — Herpes simplex may produce a follicular conjunctivitis, but more often it presents with the typical dendritic ulcer (see below).

TRIC agents — TRIC agents are no longer classified as viruses. They are intracellular parasites intermediate between viruses and *Rickettsia*. Inclusion conjunctivitis is caused by one variety. The follicular reaction is marked, but no changes occur in the cornea. The condition can be a cause of ophthalmia neonatorum in the newborn from infection via the birth canal, and in adults by sexual transmission.

In the Middle East the clinical picture of trachoma is found. In this the follicular reaction occurs mainly in the upper lid, which eventually becomes scarred and distorted. The lashes abrade the cornea and secondary infection is frequent. The cornea is invaded superiorly by a meshwork of blood vessels (pannus), which extends from the limbus with a greyish lymphocytic infiltration of the cornea, which results in scarring. Patients should be referred for treatment with local tetracycline ointment and surgical correction of the entropion and trichiasis.

Allergic conjunctivitis — Allergic conjunctivitis is usually seen in children or young adults. There may be a history of atopy with infantile eczema and asthma. It may be possible to discover an allergen such as pets or pollen.

The condition is characterized by intense irritation and mild photophobia.

Treatment with vasoconstricting drugs has little lasting effect, but sodium cromoglycate may be beneficial.

Vernal conjunctivitis — A more severe form of the condition is found in vernal conjunctivitis or spring catarrh. It occurs in the young with a characteristic seasonal pattern of exacerbations when the weather is warm and dry.

The lids are swollen and may droop (ptosis) due to the formation of papillae in the conjunctiva. This gives the typical cobblestone-like appearance when the lid is everted (**Figure 3.2**, p. 34). These changes persist even when the condition is inactive. During the active phase a mucopurulent discharge collects under the upper lids. The cornea may become very roughened and the upper limbus becomes oedematous.

Treatment with local antibiotics to control secondary infection and sodium cromoglycate may be safely given, but if there is no improvement, referral for steroid therapy is indicated. Local steroid drops can produce such rapid amelioration that there is a tendency for patients to continue treatment without proper supervision and risk developing steroid-induced glaucoma.

Episcleritis

Inflammation of the superficial tissues over the sclera is called episcleritis. This may spread to the deeper layers as scleritis.

Episcleritis is a less common cause of a painful red eye.

Symptoms and signs
The pain tends to be a dull ache and the eye may be tender to touch through the lids. The redness is usually segmental, affecting only part of the eye. The conjunctival blood vessels are dilated and there is an underlying pink blush. The lesion may be raised into a nodule (**Figure 3.3**, p. 35).

The condition is one of the 'collagen' disorders. Untreated it resolves spontaneously after 6–8 weeks, but may recur.

Treatment
Treatment with local steroid drops will usually shorten the acute phase.

Occasionally, intraocular inflammation may be present in the form of anterior uveitis, with a reduction in the vision and photophobia.

Extension to involve the sclera as scleritis is far more serious. It is seen in association with rheumatoid arthritis. The condition is more painful and requires referral for treatment with systemic steroids.

Keratitis

Inflammation of the cornea may start as conjunctivitis and spread to give rise to keratitis.

When it involves the superficial epithelial layers a superficial punctate keratitis may develop. The eye is red and gritty

The red eye

and may stain with fluorescein. There are numerous causes from infection to the dry eye of keratoconjunctivitis sicca.

Causes   Corneal ulcers may develop from infection of minor abrasions, but the most important is the dendritic ulcer.

Dendritic ulcer

The herpes simplex virus or cold sore virus causes not only the typical blisters on the lips, but also herpetic keratitis.

Presentation   The dendritic ulcer presents as a mildly red eye with slight discomfort and minimal visual problems. When stained with fluorescein the typical branching pattern is seen (**Figure 3.4**, p. 35). If left untreated the ulcer enlarges to form the amoeboid ulcer, a large irregularly shaped staining area.

Treatment   Antiviral drugs should be started immediately. Idoxuridine as ointment or drops must be given with a mydriatic. Chloramphenicol ointment should be added to counter any secondary infection.

A dendritic ulcer should clear within 6–10 days but, occasionally, longer treatment is necessary.

Often the mild initial discomfort is replaced, as the ulcer heals, by a more severe pain. The reason is that the deeper corneal stroma tends to become inflamed as the epithelium heals. This inflammation may subsequently recur, without the ulcer formation, causing a red painful eye with a hazy cornea (disciform keratitis).

Inflammation within the eye – anterior uveitis – may occur with a rise in intraocular pressure or secondary glaucoma.

Treatment of all herpetic disease should be carried out by an ophthalmic department.

The indiscriminate use of local steroid drops may result in a simple dendritic ulcer developing into such severe inflammation that the sight is lost.

As herpetic eye disease is recurrent, all patients should be warned to pay heed to the earliest symptoms and to seek immediate attention.

Iritis

The terms 'iritis', 'anterior uveitis' and 'iridocyclitis' are interchangeable. The condition consists of inflammation of the anterior portion of the uveal tract.

Cause   Iritis may be part of a generalized disorder, but more

Problems in ophthalmology

often it occurs without any other signs of systemic disease. The differentiation of the possible causes may be considered once the ocular aspects have been controlled.

Presentation
Redness. The earliest changes are seen at the limbus (ciliary injection) where a pink blush appears over the sclera. As the condition progresses the entire conjunctiva becomes involved.

Pain. This presents as an early symptom and is usually moderate to severe. It is described as a deep pain in the eye and is due to the spasm of the pupil sphincter muscles.

Photophobia. A dislike of a bright light is an early symptom. It may be noticed when watching television or when facing the head lights of oncoming traffic at night.

Poor vision. A deterioration in the level of vision is a variable feature. In 'visually aware' patients it may be the presenting symptom, while in others it may not be noticed until the condition is well established.

With a magnifying lens it may be possible to see deposits of white cells on the corneal endothelium (keratic precipitates). These are usually centrally placed and minute, but when syphilis, tuberculosis or sarcoidosis are the cause, the deposits may be much larger.

The anterior chamber contains protein, which may form into an exudate, filling the pupil.

White cells may sediment to the bottom of the anterior chamber forming a horizontal whitish line (hypopyon). The pupil tends to be small and the iris becomes adherent to the lens forming posterior synechiae, which are more obvious when the pupil is dilated (**Figure 3.5**, p. 36).

If the intraocular pressure rises, the cornea may become waterlogged, losing its lustre and normal clarity.

The patient should be referred for treatment.

Treatment
The inflammation is controlled with local steroid drops. These are given every 2 hours or even hourly when the condition is acute. The frequency is gradually reduced as the condition improves.

It is sometimes necessary to give subconjunctival injections of steroids in the very severe cases.

The pupil is dilated with a mydriatic drop. In mild cases cyclopentolate 1% (Mydrilate) or homatropine 1–2% produces adequate dilation of the pupil, but in the more severe cases atropine 1% is required.

Secondary glaucoma is treated with acetazolamide (Diamox) or dichlorphenamide (Daranide or Oratrol).

The red eye

Acute glaucoma

Acute glaucoma is one of the most dramatic diseases that can present to the medical practitioner.

The condition, which normally starts in one eye, tends to affect the middle-aged, longsighted, female.

The intraocular pressure rises due to obstruction of the drainage mechanism by the apposition of the iris to the cornea. This tends to occur in the eye with a shallow anterior chamber when the pupil is dilated.

Presentation Subacute attacks may precede the typical acute episode. The patient complains of mild pain in the eye with blurring of vision. The attacks tend to occur when the light is poor and the pupils dilate. On direct questioning, haloes of coloured light may be noticed around lights due to the presence of fluid within the cornea. The attacks usually settle overnight as the pupils constrict during sleep.

Subacute attacks may occur for several months before an acute episode.

Acute glaucoma develops over several hours. The most noticeable features are severe prostrating pain and loss of vision. The pain, which starts in the eye, may radiate over the head. Its severity is such that patients may develop profuse vomiting, suggesting an abdominal cause. The loss of vision is acute with a rapid reduction to no perception of light.

Signs The eye is markedly injected and the cornea hazy due to the fluid forced into it. The haziness of the cornea may mask the changes inside the eye. The anterior is very shallow and the pupil semidilated, fixed and vertically oval (**Figure 3.6**, p. 36). The details of the iris appear indistinct but the iris may show a spiral arrangement. When the intraocular pressure is felt by the digital method it is stony-hard compared with the fellow eye.

Treatment *Immediate referral* is necessary to save the sight. If this is impossible miotic drops will constrict the pupil and open the angle of the anterior chamber.

Pilocarpine 4% drops should be given every 5 minutes for half an hour and then hourly for 6 hours.

Acetazolamide 500 mg is given intramuscularly to diminish the normal aqueous secretion.

Pilocarpine 2% drops should also be instilled in the normal eye to prevent a similar closure of the angle.

When the immediate rise in pressure has been controlled, surgery is required to prevent a recurrence of the acute attack. A peripheral iridectomy removes a small part of the iris so that aqueous can drain through the hole that is formed rather than the pupil. This prevents a build-up of pressure behind the iris which forces it forward to close the angle.

Prophylactic iridectomy is also performed on the normal eye.

4 The external eye

Introduction – Lids – Conjunctiva

Introduction

Lesions affecting the lids and the front of the eye are usually the cause of cosmetic embarrassment, sometimes of discomfort, but rarely of visual disturbance.

Lids

Blepharitis

This inflammation of the lids is common and tiresome to both patient and doctor because of its recurrent nature. Two types are found – squamous and ulcerative.

Squamous blepharitis

Squamous blepharitis may occur in the presence of dandruff of the scalp. The lid margins are red and irritate and scales of dry skin are caught on the lashes. Occasionally, the conjunctiva may also be inflamed.

Treatment

The scales on the lashes should be rubbed off and a non-steroid ointment applied to the lid margins. Oxyphenbutazone with chloramphenicol (Tanderil Chloramphenicol) is palliative but not curative and the patient should be warned of the chronic nature of the condition.

Ulcerative blepharitis

Infection of the lash follicles can cause multiple small ulcers of the lid margin. This can be treated with local antibiotic ointment.

Problems in ophthalmology

Stye

This is a localized staphylococcal infection of the lash follicle.

Treatment — Treatment is usually not required unless there is a tendency to recurrences. This happens in young children probably from reinfection of an adjacent lash follicle. A course of 10 days' local antibiotic drops and ointment may be necessary.

Chalazion

The meibomian glands lie in the tarsal plates of the lids. If the secretion becomes inspissated the gland enlarges and the swelling becomes visible under the skin (**Figure 4.1**, p. 37).

Treatment — The contents of the gland may liquify and the cyst resolve spontaneously. This can be helped by local antibiotic drops to counter any infection.

If the cyst remains, the centre undergoes a granulomatous change and incision and curettage are then required.

Herpes zoster ophthalmicus

This viral infection can involve the fifth cranial nerve to produce the typical clinical picture (**Figure 4.2**, p. 37).

Early symptoms — Early diagnosis can be made by the unilateral pain that occurs over the forehead for 4–5 days before the appearance of the rash. Treatment at this stage with a solution of idoxuridine (Herpid), although expensive, may help to limit the skin changes if started early enough.

Rash — The rash involves the area of distribution of the ophthalmic division of the fifth cranial nerve with blistering, scabbing and finally scarring of the skin.

The patient looks and feels wretched, but there is always a marked improvement when the skin eruption heals. In the early stages it is impossible to examine the eye itself because of swelling of the lids – if, however, blisters involve the tip of the nose, there is every chance that the eye will also be affected. Local antibiotic drops should be instilled while the swelling persists.

Eye involvement — Ocular involvement can be serious and the eye should be carefully examined in every case.

The conjunctiva may be red, with corneal erosions shown by fluorescein staining.

Iritis may be present with secondary glaucoma.

Rarely there is involvement of the optic nerve with optic

The external eye

atrophy and extraocular muscle weakness, which results in double vision.

Treatment   All cases with ocular involvement should be referred. Iritis and raised intraocular pressure must be treated with local steroids and systemic antiglaucoma therapy.

Long-term management may be necessary as the anaesthetic cornea is prone to ulceration. In addition, post-herpetic neuralgia may persist for months or even years, with the forehead and scalp exquisitely tender. Light touch or even a wind can produce very unpleasant sensations so that it becomes impossible to comb or brush the hair or even wear a hat.

Entropion

Cause   This condition is seen in the elderly when the lower lid margin is turned inwards. It is caused by spasm of the fibres of the orbicularis muscle (**Figure 4.3**, p. 38). The eye feels gritty as the lashes rub on the cornea. This tends to produce more spasm and a vicious circle is started.

Treatment   First-aid treatment can be given by strapping the lower lid to the cheek (**Figure 4.4**, p. 38) and giving antibiotic ointment, but surgical correction is ultimately necessary.

The upper lid may be turned in when the eye is affected by trachoma. Scarring of the conjunctival surface of the lid results in entropion, so that the lashes abrade the already inflamed cornea. The condition can only be corrected by surgery.

Ectropion

Here the lower lid margin is turned away from the eye (**Figure 4.5**, p. 39). The condition is most commonly seen in old age when
Cause   the orbicularis muscle becomes atonic. The sagging lid prevents normal drainage of tears as the punctum is pulled away from the eyeball. The stagnant tears become infected and the conjunctival lining of the lid becomes thickened and red.

Treatment   While local antibiotic drops or ointment may relieve any infection, the repositioning of the lid can only be done by surgery. The patient should be instructed not to wipe any tears away with a downward movement as this tends to worsen the condition. Rather he or she should wipe upwards.

Tumours of the lids

Numerous lumps can appear on and around the lids, some of which are unsightly while others are dangerous.

Problems in ophthalmology

Clear cyst
: The lid margin is the site for clear cysts arising from sweat glands. These can be punctured with a needle and rarely re-form.

Sebaceous cyst
: Sebaceous cysts are common and can be removed when very small without local anaesthesia.

Papillomata
: Papillomata may be left if small, but ultimately require surgical excision.

Xanthelasma
: In xanthelasma, lipid deposits at the medial ends of upper and lower lids appear as flat yellowish-white areas. Excision is necessary and serum lipids should be investigated.

Rodent ulcer

Presentation
: The basal cell carcinoma of the lid is a malignant tumour that does not spread to regional lymph glands, but can cause extensive local damage if left untreated. The condition presents in middle age with a small nodule that gradually increases in size over several months (**Figure 4.6**, p. 39). The surface tends to break down and may bleed. Some of the lesions have a well-marked edge while others are more invasive and it is difficult to define the limit of their extension.

Treatment
: Local excision produces a cure rate of over 95%. When the lid margin is involved a full thickness wedge of the lid must be excised. This should be carried out by an ophthalmic surgeon, who is used to lid reconstruction.

Radiotherapy can produce cure rates similar to those achieved by surgical excision. However, the complications limit its use to the elderly patient who cannot withstand major plastic reconstruction of the lids. Scarring and telangiectasia are common complications.

Conjunctiva

Subconjunctival haemorrhage

This occurs spontaneously in the elderly arteriosclerotic patients and is commonly noticed on waking. Occasionally it may follow lifting or straining.

Presentation
: It is rarely associated with any pain or discomfort. The bright-red blood covers a variable area of the white of the eye and looks more serious than it really is.

It retains its bright colour while being absorbed, as the haemoglobin does not break down.

Complete absorption usually occurs within 10–14 days without treatment. The patient should be reassured that the condition is only on the surface and that the blood cannot leak into the eye.

If the condition is recurrent, the blood pressure should be

taken and a blood count performed together with the tests for any haemorrhagic diathesis. These are nearly always normal, confirming that the condition is caused by leakage from a weakened arteriosclerotic vessel. Occasionally, cautery to an area of conjunctival vessels may prevent recurrence when the haemorrhages keep appearing in the same segment.

Conjunctival cysts

These appear suddenly as transparent swellings on the sclera, varying in size from less than a pin head to several millimetres in diameter.

Treatment is usually unnecessary, but they can be lanced with a needle if they enlarge. A topical anaesthetic, oxybuprocaine (Minims Benoxinate), is used and the cyst is incised.

Pinguecula

This degenerative condition is a common cause of painless redness of a segment of the sclera.

Presentation The lesions appear as small whitish-yellow patches like fatty deposits on the sclera adjacent to the cornea in the 3-o'clock and 9-o'clock positions (**Figure 4.7**, p. 40). After the age of 40 most patients show the lesions which are completely benign.

Treatment Occasionally the eye becomes inflamed around the lesion and treatment with local astringent drops (Zincfrin) or even a local steroid may be necessary.

Pterygium

This is a more serious degenerative condition of the conjunctiva, which is related to exposure to a hot dusty atmosphere.

Presentation The lesion appears on the nasal or temporal side of the cornea as a greyish nodule with a leash of blood vessels spreading onto the conjunctiva (**Figure 4.8**, p. 40). It extends gradually across the cornea and will impair the vision if the centre is reached. Bouts of acute redness and discomfort occur intermittently.

Treatment Local steroid drops will suppress the acute attacks of redness. If the lesion is threatening the vision, then surgical excision is indicated. The recurrence rate is high and, occasionally, radiotherapy may be needed to suppress further corneal involvement.

5 The internal eye

Examination of the inner eye – Alteration in pigment – Toxoplasmosis – Toxocara – Opaque nerve fibres

Examination of the inner eye

Introduction — The ability to use an ophthalmoscope competently is essential if the examination of the inner eye is to be attempted. Every effort should be made to examine both eyes of as many patients as possible, for it is only then that the wide spectrum of normality will be appreciated. When it is convenient the pupils should be dilated.

Vitreous — The normal vitreous is an optically transparent medium, but it is not unusual to find minute dots or strands after the third

Floaters — decade. These may be symptomless or may appear to the patient as cobwebs or flies which swing across the vision as the eye moves.

Vitreous detachment — Occasionally more marked 'floaters' are noticed together with flashing lights. The vitreous changes may be more noticeable and a complete ringlike opacity may be found. This is due to a posterior detachment of the vitreous from its normal

Floaters and flashes — attachment around the optic disc. Referral for a full retinal assessment is advisable, especially if the patient is shortsighted, because of the greater risk of retinal tears and detachment.

Fundus — The colour of the normal fundus varies between the races and the different age groups, and is related to the density and the distribution of pigment in the pigment epithelium and the underlying choroid. In the coloured races, the colour ranges from dark red to coffee-brown or even grey (**Figure 5.1**, p. 73),

Problems in ophthalmology

while in the white-skinned the fundus appears bright orange (**Figure 5.2**, p. 73). In childhood the colour is at its most brilliant, but with increasing age the intensity fades.

The choroidal vessels may be readily visible especially in myopia and are distinguished from the retinal vessels by being much broader and more numerous.

Occasionally pigment may be condensed between the choroidal vessels to give the tigroid or tessellated fundus.

Macula   The macula lies temporal to the disc, and may be marked by an oval reflection of light slightly larger than the disc diameter with a bright pinpoint of light at its foveal centre. It tends to be slightly darker in colour than the surrounding retina and is avascular.

The disc   The optic disc is the site where the retinal nerve fibres leave the eye to form the optic nerve. There are no light-sensitive cells on the disc, which is represented in the field of vision by the blind spot.

Normal disc   The normal disc is round, with a slightly pink rim and a central depression – 'the physiological cup' (**Figure 5.2**). Considerable variations can exist, but the appearance of the discs is remarkably similar in both eyes.

Hypermetropic disc   In the hypermetropic eye the disc looks small, greyish-pink and slightly raised (pseudopapilloedema). The physiological cupping may be small or even absent. Light reflected from the surrounding retina gives the appearance of watered silk.

Myopic disc   In contrast, the myopic disc appears larger and more pale than normal (**Figure 5.3**, p. 74). A crescent of exposed sclera, choroid or pigment epithelium is often present on the temporal side, giving either a white, pink of black 'new moon' crescent to the edge of the disc. The physiological cup varies in size and depth. The diameter is usually between a quarter and half the disc diameter. The depth may be quite marked and yet not signify any pathological change.

The retinal vessels   The retinal vessels emerge from the centre or nasal side of the physiological cup and divide to supply the four quarters of the retina. Occasionally a cilio-retinal artery leaves the temporal edge of the disc to supply the macular area.

The retinal arteries appear narrower than the veins and are a bright-red colour, with a sharp light reflex. The veins are wider and darker than the arteries and venous pulsation may be seen at the disc. This has little clinical significance except that pulsation does not occur when the cerebrospinal pressure is raised. Therefore, if venous pulsations are seen the intracranial pressure is normal.

The internal eye

Alteration in pigment

Pigment clumps

Isolated marks of pigment may occur throughout the fundus. These appear as coal-black sharply defined spots which may be solitary or grouped together like the tracks of an animal.

Naevus

The benign choroidal naevus is symptomless and appears as a slate-grey patch usually about the same size as the disc. The edge is indistinct and the tumour is flat (**Figure 5.4**, p. 74). No treatment is necessary for this congenital lesion, but if it appears raised the patient should be referred for fluorescein angiography and serial photography to differentiate it from a malignant melanoma.

Malignant melanoma

The malignant melanoma occurs in the fifth decade either as a chance finding on routine ophthalmoscopy or because of the appearance of a defect in the visual field.

Findings   The lesion starts as a flat pale area, but rapidly increases in size to become raised above the surrounding retina. The colour varies from a light greyish-brown to a dark brown depending on the degree of pigmentation (**Figure 5.5**, p. 75). The more malignant tumours tend to have less pigment and may appear mottled.

The tumour tends to be highly vascular, and fragile new vessels appear on its surface. These can be the cause of small haemorrhages into the retina or even into the vitreous.

An area of retina below the tumour may be detached due to a collection of subretinal serous fluid. Occasionally this inferior detachment may be separated from the tumour by an area of normal flat retina.

The tumour gradually increases in size and the central vision fails when the macula becomes involved. Eventually the entire vitreous cavity is replaced by tumour and glaucoma develops.

Treatment   The operation of enucleation of the globe is advisable for tumours larger than 15 mm diameter. (The optic disc is 1.5 mm diameter.) For smaller tumours, however, observation combined with radiotherapy or photocoagulation is replacing surgical removal.

Problems in ophthalmology

Drusen

These common lesions are also known as 'colloid bodies'. They appear as round yellow spots occurring singly or in groups scattered throughout the fundus (**Figure 5.6**, p. 75). Although increasing with age they do not affect the vision. In the peripheral retina the spots may be outlined by pigment to give the appearance of cobblestones.

Toxoplasmosis

This protozoal disease is caused by an intracellular parasite and has a widespread distribution in man. Although nearly 30% of the population over 50 years old in England can be shown to have positive serological tests, the infection is usually subclinical and symptoms and signs are absent.

Presentation   The disease is acquired congenitally from the mother who has a subclinical infection. This may result in miscarriage or the child may be born with signs of neuro-ectodermal involvement. Hydrocephalus, with convulsions, occurs and X-rays of the skull show calcification over the cerebral cortex and basal ganglia.

The ocular disease may be found during the first 6 months or may only be discovered on routine examination years later. In the active phase the visual acuity is reduced due to the haziness of the vitreous.

Findings   The lesions may be solitary or multiple and can affect one or both eyes. They occur most often at the posterior pole of the globe, particularly at the macula.

The lesions are pearly-white with deeply pigmented sharp edges. They vary in size from half the disc diameter to several times the width of the disc (**Figure 5.7**, p. 76).

If the macula is involved a squint or nystagmus may be present.

Management   When the lesions do not involve the macula and are obviously inactive with no overlying vitreous haziness, no treatment is required.

When the visual acuity is affected or a squint is present, referral for full ophthalmic assessment is necessary.

The diagnosis of the condition can be confirmed with serological tests – the dye test and the complement fixation test.

Treatment   The condition is very resistant to all treatment. Local and systemic steroids help to suppress the inflammatory signs and may be aided by sulphadiazine.

The internal eye

Toxocara

This common intestinal parasite of dogs may cause systemic and ocular complications.

Presentation
The ingested ova enter the blood vessels or lymphatics of the intestinal wall and are widely distributed throughout the body to produce the syndrome of visceral larva migrans (eosinophilia, hepatomegaly and intermittent fever).

Chance involvement of the eye may produce a discrete granuloma at or near the macula (**Figure 5.8**, p. 76). It is white and may mimic a retinoblastoma. A chronic endophthalmitis with redness of the eye, lowered visual acuity and haziness of the vitreous can also occur.

Management
The diagnosis of toxocara in the early stages can be confirmed by an eosinophilia of 3–12%. The retinal granuloma does not enlarge like retinoblastoma, nor is calcification visible on X-rays.

No specific treatment is available, but steroids – either systemic or local – may be of use when there is chronic inflammation. The most effective action against the disease is by separating young babies from puppies and by regular deworming of adult dogs.

Opaque nerve fibres

Medullation of the optic nerve fibres usually stops at the disc, but occasionally the retinal nerve fibres are also involved.

The appearance is characteristic with a white area extending from the edge of the disc (**Figure 5.9**, p. 77). Its size is variable and its edge is feathery. The blind spot may be enlarged, but otherwise no visual problems occur.

6 Sudden loss of vision

Introduction – Migraine – Amaurosis fugax – Retinal artery occlusion – Temporal arteritis – Retinal vein occlusion – Vitreous haemorrhage – Retinal detachment

Introduction

Sudden loss of vision is one of the most alarming symptoms that can happen to a patient and, unlike slow loss of vision which may pass unnoticed, a sudden deterioration is rarely missed.

The timing of the visual loss may be over a few minutes or can extend to several hours. It may involve only part of the visual field – as following a retinal detachment – or the entire field after occlusion of the central retinal artery.

The correct early diagnosis and appropriate referral is of vital importance if those diseases that are treatable are not to be left to become permanently blinding conditions.

The conditions most likely to present to the general practitioner are as follows.

Loss within minutes	(1) Migraine (2) Amaurosis fugax (3) Retinal artery occlusion	} vision lost within minutes
Loss within minutes or hours	(4) Temporal arteritis (5) Retinal vein occlusion (6) Vitreous haemorrhage (7) Retinal detachment	} vision lost within minutes or hours.

Problems in ophthalmology

Migraine

The condition of migraine is included here as it is a common cause for sudden loss or disturbance of vision and may be confused with amaurosis fugax and retinal detachment.

Presentation Migraine is a familial disorder characterized by recurrent attacks of headache, which are usually unilateral and may be associated with photophobia, nausea and vomiting. The headache may be preceded by prodromal symptoms such as depression or even euphoria, and an aura which is usually visual.

It is the visual aura of the first attack that worries the patient and may confuse the doctor.

Visual aura The patient may be unable to describe the visual symptoms accurately, but more often there is a distinct pattern.

Flashing lights are seen in the peripheral field of vision of one or both eyes, usually on the temporal side. These may appear as sparks or flashes of lightning and are frequently in the primary colours. Over a period of minutes the area of the lights expands towards the centre of vision, but the central vision is usually spared. In some patients the reverse pattern is seen. A small blind area is noted to one side of the point of fixation. This area gradually enlarges and is edged by a zigzag pattern of coloured light (the fortification spectrum). The lights eventually reach the peripheral field and disappear.

The visual aura lasts up to half an hour, while the blind area or scotoma usually takes a little longer to recover. Very rarely the field defect may persist. The aura may be accompanied by other sensory disturbances with paraesthesiae of the upper limbs and face.

The headache The intermittent headache is usually unilateral although it may spread to involve the whole head. It is typically throbbing in character and made worse by any exertion. It is associated with photophobia so that the patient prefers a darkened room. Nausea and vomiting are common and these symptoms may in fact relieve the headache.

The headache persists until the following day, although the patient may still feel unwell after it has cleared.

Ophthalmoplegia Very rarely migraine may be associated with paresis of the extraocular muscles, usually by involvement of the third cranial nerve.

Management The common occurrence of migraine often results in the doctor showing a lack of overt interest. Sympathetic reassurance by a visibly interested doctor can, however, make a great difference to the successful management of this debilitating

Sudden loss of vision

condition. Certain precipitating factors may be identified and avoided. Foods containing tyramine may initiate an attack, which may also occur with hunger, stress and, occasionally, release from stress.

Symptomatic treatment for the headache and vomiting may be needed. Because of vomiting and reduced peristalsis, absorption of medication may be affected so that sublingual or rectal administration may be necessary.

Ergotamine forms the basis of most available preparations, but care should be taken that habituation does not develop. A single dose of ergotamine should be taken as early as possible in the attack, but not repeated.

Prophylactic treatment may be needed when there are severe or repeated attacks. Clonidine (Dixarit), pizotifen (Sanomigran) and methysergide (Deseril) may be used – with caution, as all have side-effects and some contraindications.

Amaurosis fugax

Amaurosis fugax or 'fleeting blindness' is marked by sudden loss of vision due to embolization of the retinal arteries. The importance of the condition is its association with transient ischaemic attacks of the brain.

Presentation — The patient complains of a sudden painless loss of vision, the extent of which will depend on the retinal vessel involved. Total loss of vision occurs if the central retinal artery is blocked. When either the upper or lower division is affected, the visual loss will be in the corresponding lower or upper field. The loss is often described as a shutter or curtain covering the vision from above or below.

There is complete recovery from the visual loss which only lasts 2–3 minutes so that the patient is rarely seen in the acute phase.

Findings — It is necessary to dilate the pupils of these patients to obtain a satisfactory view of the retinal vasculature.

It may then be possible to locate the embolus, the site of obstruction being estimated from the description of the visual loss.

Cholesterol emboli arise from an atheromatous plaque in the internal carotid artery. The embolus appears as a glistening crystal, often appearing larger than the vessel wall. It may become impacted at an arterial bifurcation or at the junction of artery and vein (**Figure 6.1**, p. 78).

Problems in ophthalmology

Platelet emboli appear as small white plugs in the artery, which tend to break up and pass into more peripheral vessels.

Management
The origin of the emboli should be sought by examination of the heart for signs of rheumatic or ischaemic heart disease and listening over the carotid arteries for any bruits.

If there is a history of anaesthesia or muscle weakness implying cerebral ischaemia, the patient should be referred for investigation. Carotid endarterectomy may be indicated in some cases while others require anticoagulation to lessen the risk of stroke. The use of aspirin and dipyridamole (Persantin) can also help by decreasing platelet adhesiveness.

Retinal artery occlusion

Obstruction of the central retinal artery or of one of its branches produces a sudden and usually irreversible loss of vision.

Presentation
The onset of the visual loss is similar to that found in amaurosis fugax. Involvement of the central artery causes complete loss, obstruction to an upper or lower division produces an altitudinal loss, while blockage of the temporal or nasal branches results in a sectorial loss in the appropriate quadrant of the field of vision.

Findings
The area of affected retina shows signs of anoxia within a few hours. The retina becomes white and thickened by oedema, the arteries are thread-like and the disc may be swollen. When the central artery is affected the retinal oedema masks the usual red reflex from the choroid except at the fovea, which shows as a bright cherry-red spot (**Figure 6.2**, p. 78).

When only part of the retina is involved there is a sharp demarcation between the healthy pink retina and the white ischaemic retina (**Figure 6.3**, p. 79).

Management
Immediate action is required if the vision is to be restored. Intravenous acetazolamide (Diamox) 500 mg should be given and the eye massaged to attempt to dislodge any emboli.

In some centres intravenous dexamethasone 10 mg is also given to treat those cases caused by temporal arteritis.

All cases should be sent immediately to the nearest hospital where ophthalmic assessment is available.

Temporal arteritis

Temporal or giant cell arteritis is a generalized condition affecting those over the age of 55, particularly women. Half of the

Sudden loss of vision

cases suffer ocular involvement which, if not treated, can result in blindness in both eyes.

Presentation
The general symptoms of the condition are insidious so that the diagnosis is often only made when the catastrophic ocular complications occur. There is weight loss and general malaise. The condition may present as polymyalgia rheumatica with pain in the limbs, particularly the muscles.

When the temporal arteries become involved the scalp is tender to touch, so that it is painful to brush the hair or lie on a pillow. Chewing may be painful when the facial arteries are affected.

The diagnosis is confirmed by the high ESR (100 mm/hour) and further evidence may be gained from biopsy of a tender portion of the temporal artery.

The visual problems may be heralded by attacks of amaurosis fugax or of vague mistiness with photopsia which may be dismissed as migraine. Eventually, obstruction of the central retinal artery occurs with sudden complete loss of sight.

Management
Immediate intravenous dexamethasone 10 mg should be given and the patient transferred at once to hospital. The condition is then treated with long-term prednisolone, the dosage being adjusted according to the level of the ESR.

Retinal vein occlusion

As with arterial obstruction, venous occlusion may affect either the central retinal vessel or one of its tributaries.

Presentation
The visual deterioration is not so dramatic as that found with arterial obstruction. The loss may first be noticed on waking. The patient is usually over the age of 60 and has hypertension. Some have diabetes, while others have a blood dyscrasia which increases the viscosity of the blood.

Findings
The typical picture is one of widespread haemorrhages with dilated tortuous veins. The haemorrhages most easily visible are the so-called flame-shaped variety with a streaky feathery pattern where the blood has leaked into the nerve fibre layer (**Figure 6.4**, p. 79). In the deeper layers of the retina are more discrete round-shaped haemorrhages. Spots of soft or cotton-wool exudates occur where infarction of the retina occurs. The dilated veins seem to disappear as the vessels loop in and out of the swollen retina. Haemorrhages and swelling of the disc can also occur.

When a branch retinal vein is occluded the retinal changes are confined to the quadrant drained by the vessel. This most commonly occurs in the superior temporal vein (**Figure 6.5**, p. 80). Hypertension is found more commonly in those with branch vein occlusion than those with central retinal vein occlusion.

Management The blood pressure is recorded and urine is tested for sugar. The patient should be referred for ophthalmic assessment and follow-up because of the possible complications.

Central retinal vein occlusion may be associated with pre-existing chronic simple glaucoma and 20% of cases develop thrombotic glaucoma with neovascularization of the iris.

Photocoagulation of the retina may help to prevent this secondary glaucoma, which tends to develop within 3 months. Branch retinal vein occlusion may cause severe visual loss without obvious changes in the retina. This is due to fluid leaking from vessels adjacent to the macular area. Neovascularization of the retina may also occur and rupture of these fragile new vessels results in vitreous haemorrhage.

Drug therapy is currently used for both types of vein occlusion. Anticoagulation may have a place, together with aspirin and dipyridamole (Persantin) to reduce platelet adhesiveness.

Vitreous haemorrhage

Causes Vitreous haemorrhage produces a sudden dimming of the sight over a period of minutes. Most often the blood leaks either from the fragile vessels in an area of neovascularization seen in diabetes and branch retinal vein occlusion, or from a torn retinal vessel associated with a retinal detachment.

Findings In the older age group the red reflex may be completely lost and the vision reduced to hand movements or less, as the blood is evenly distributed throughout the vitreous. In the younger patient with a more solid vitreous the blood is seen as black streaks against the red reflex.

Management Every case of vitreous haemorrhage should be assumed to originate from a retinal tear until proved otherwise. The patient should be referred the same day for inpatient supervision. Bed rest will allow the blood to absorb so that a satisfactory view of the fundus can be obtained.

Occasionally, a vitreous haemorrhage does not absorb and surgical removal by vitrectomy is indicated. This may be preceded by ultrasound investigation to determine if an underlying detachment is present.

Sudden loss of vision

Retinal detachment

Retinal detachment occurs when the layer of rods and cones becomes separated from the underlying epithelium, which is normally responsible for the nutrition of the light-sensitive cells. The cause is a tear in the retina allowing fluid to leak behind it. This occurs most commonly in myopic eyes or following trauma.

Presentation

Floaters and flashes

The patient notices a sudden shower of black spots or 'cobwebs' floating in the vision associated with small sparks or flashes of light in the peripheral field of vision. The appearance is more dramatic than, and differs from, the type of spot which moves with the eye and which is occasionally noticed by most people, especially myopic patients. The floaters are caused by vitreous haemorrhage, and the flashes by stimulation of the retina by traction from the vitreous.

Visual loss

A curtain or shadow may appear to cover part of the sight and may extend to involve the central vision, if the macula is detached.

Findings

The visual acuity may be normal if the macula is unaffected, but may be reduced if there is much haemorrhage into the vitreous. On examining the fundus the detached retina appears normal when the detachment is very shallow, but grey when there is a large quantity of subretinal fluid (**Figure 6.6**, p. 80). Occasionally, the retina may balloon forwards into the vitreous. The surface may have a rippled appearance which undulates with the movement of the eye.

If the blood vessels are followed from the disc they appear to darken when the detached retina is reached.

It may be possible to see the cause of the detachment if the pupil is dilated, but it may take several days before the vitreous is sufficiently clear of blood to see any retinal holes. The holes are usually found opposite the quadrant in which the flashes of light were noticed and are most common in the upper temporal quadrant.

Management

The patient should be referred the same day for admission. Detachments of the upper half of the retina create a greater risk as gravity causes the subretinal fluid to track down, so increasing the detachment. This may then involve a previously normal macula.

Surgical treatment

Surgical repositioning of the retina is achieved by indentation of the sclera from outside by the application of pieces of silicone sponge. Occasionally, the eye is encircled by a band of silicone rubber. Adhesion is produced by cryotherapy which causes an inflammatory reaction within the retina.

Problems in ophthalmology

Inpatient treatment for detachment surgery is usually for 1–2 weeks. The patient is mobilized soon after surgery and can usually return to sedentary work in 6 weeks.

Prophylactic treatment
Prophylactic treatment as day cases can be given to weak areas in the retina using photocoagulation or cryotherapy.

7 Slow loss of vision

Introduction – Cataract – Chronic glaucoma – Macular degeneration

Introduction

There are three main causes for a gradual deterioration in the level of vision, listed below. These usually occur over several weeks or even months.

(1) Cataract
(2) Chronic glaucoma
(3) Macular degeneration.

All three are diseases of the middle-aged or elderly and together they account for nearly two thirds of the patients registered as blind in the United Kingdom.

Cataract

Definition
A cataract is produced when there is an alteration in the optical clarity of the lens.
This is usually associated with a change in the lens so that it becomes opaque (cortical cataract) (**Figure 7.1**, p. 89). Occasionally the nucleus of the lens becomes harder and more optically dense (nuclear sclerosis) (**Figure 7.2**, p. 89).

Presentation
The sight fails gradually over a period of months or even years and both distance vision and near vision are affected. The level of illumination becomes critical so that too little light makes seeing impossible, while too much causes dazzle. Mono-

Problems in ophthalmology

cular double vision may be troublesome and must always be differentiated from double vision seen with the two eyes. If the double vision disappears when one eye is shut, then it is associated with a squint. Haloes appear around lights at night, so that night driving may become dangerous. The colour of these haloes is usually white; this distinguishes them from those seen in acute glaucoma, which are rainbow coloured.

Management A cataract should be removed when the vision has fallen to a level which prevents the patient from continuing with his normal everyday tasks. Thus the timing for surgery for a watchmaker will be much earlier than that needed to manage the cataract in the elderly patient.

Occasionally it is necessary to remove a cataract that has become hypermature. The hypermature cataract is like a bag of fluid which can easily rupture, releasing lens protein into the anterior chamber. The lens protein can produce a marked inflammatory reaction or may block the drainage angle and so cause secondary glaucoma.

When a cataract is first diagnosed it may be less alarming to the patient to call it a cloudiness or haze in the lens, rather than use the word 'cataract' with all its connotations of blindness.

Referral for glasses The patient should be referred to an optician for a test for glasses which may restore the vision to its previous level.

Advice for early stages of cataract The patient should be warned that bright light shining directly onto the eye will impair the vision. When possible a hat with a brim or a tennis eyeshield should be worn to protect the eye from direct sunlight. This is particularly troublesome in spring and autumn when the sun is low in the sky. A lightly tinted distance glass may also help. Indoors, the patient should sit with the light behind him keeping his face in the shadow. Ceiling lights are best avoided. When watching television the only light in front of the patient should be from the television set. When the patient is reading or sewing, the light should be as close as convenient and should shine from behind the patient over the shoulders. Glare from paper, particularly when shiny, can severely reduce the reading ability. This may be overcome by placing a sheet of matt black card over the page with a slit of 2 × 15 cm cut in it through which to view the print. This prevents reflection of unwanted light from the remainder of the page from striking the eye. Alternatively, half the page may be covered with the black card.

Rate of visual deterioration The rate at which the visual acuity falls will depend on the position of the cataract. The silhouette of the lens changes can

Sudden loss of vision

be seen against the red reflex using the ophthalmoscope at a distance of 30 cm.

If the shadows appear like the spokes of a wheel, a cortical cataract is present (**Figure 7.3**, p. 90). Here the vision may remain good as long as the centre of the lens is unaffected.

If only the centre of the lens is affected, the vision tends to fall rapidly as the opacity lies on the line of vision (**Figure 7.4**, p. 90).

If the centre of the lens appears clear, but it is difficult to focus on the retina, nuclear sclerosis is present. With more minus lenses on the ophthalmoscope the retinal details will become visible. The vision can similarly be maintained by gradually increasing the strength of the spectacles to compensate for the changing power of the patient's own lens.

Timing of hospital referral

When the visual acuity has fallen to 6/18 the patient should be referred for hospital assessment. At this level it is still possible to obtain a good view of the macular area. This is important, because signs of degenerative change may make future surgery impracticable.

If the macula appears healthy the patient may continue to attend for routine refraction until such time as he or she is unable to cope.

Unilateral cataract

Cataract is usually a bilateral condition, although initially one eye only may be affected. Much confusion surrounds the apparent refusal of surgeons to operate when only one eye is involved.

The explanation lies in the problems associated with the correction of the vision following cataract removal from one eye (unilateral aphakia). The vision can be restored using spectacles, contact lenses or an intraocular implant (see also below, p. 71).

Spectacle lenses need to be strong (+ 12 dioptres) and are therefore also thick and unattractive. Unfortunately a magnified image is produced, in the eye which has been operated on, which cannot be fused by the brain with the normal-sized image of the other eye.

Contact lenses do not produce the same magnifying effect, but they are not always suitable for the elderly patient who finds the handling of the lens too difficult. The lens must be inserted each morning and removed again in the evening.

Continuous-wear soft contact lenses are a possible alternative as the patient wears the lens all the time. However the lens and the eye must be examined frequently and this entails repeated visits to the ophthalmologist.

Surgical treatment

Cataract extraction can be performed under local or general anaesthesia. The patient is admitted either 1 or 2 days preoperatively so that the general health can be assessed if a general anaesthetic is to be used. Coughing in the 'chesty' patient can cause postoperative complications so that it may be advisable to operate on these cases during the summer months. Preoperative conjunctival swabs may be taken if the eyes appear sticky, but usually local antibiotic drops are given without resorting to bacterial cultures.

Two methods of cataract surgery are practised.

Intracapsular extraction Intracapsular extraction is the routine procedure for senile cataracts. The entire lens and its capsule are removed, by rupturing the zonular fibres that attach the lens to the ciliary muscle. For this a large wound extending around one third of the limbus is made.

Extracapsular extraction Extracapsular extraction is the method of choice for younger patients in whom the zonular fibres are very tough. Rupture of these fibres causes excessive traction on the peripheral retina with the risk of producing a retinal tear and detachment.

The extracapsular technique involves the incision of the capsule followed by the aspiration of the lens protein. The procedure can be carried out through a small corneal incision using a narrow gauge aspiration technique or phako-emulsification.

Postoperative management After either method of cataract removal the patient is mobilized on the day following surgery. The eye is kept padded for 4–5 days, after which dark glasses or temporary aphakic spectacles are worn.

The patient may be discharged within the week after the intracapsular method, or sooner when only a small corneal wound has been made.

Instructions are given to avoid stooping, straining or lifting anything heavy. The operation causes remarkably little pain, so that the patient may be tempted to do more than he or she should before the wound has healed.

For sedentary occupations there is little risk to the eye after 6 weeks and the patient may then resume normal activities. For

Sudden loss of vision

those engaged in more strenuous activities it is prudent not to return to work before 8 weeks.

Correction of aphakia

Spectacles have been the traditional method for the correction of aphakia for many years, but are now being replaced by the contact lens and the intraocular implant.

Each method has its advantages and drawbacks to the patient, and its supporters among ophthalmic surgeons. Whichever method is chosen, the patient must still use reading glasses since the eye is no longer able to accommodate.

Spectacles   In addition to the magnification effect already mentioned, the thick lenses used in spectacles produce considerable distortion. Although the visual acuity is normal through the centre of the lens, when the patient turns to look through the peripheral area his view of life becomes very disturbing. Horizontal lines appear to curve upwards at the end, while doorways become alarmingly narrow. People and objects may seem to disappear in the peripheral field of vision only to reappear suddenly in the centre of the vision.

Due to the magnifying effect, objects are thought to be nearer than they really are. The assessment of distance is difficult, and many a cup of tea will be poured inadvertently into the saucer.

With perseverence these problems tend to settle down. However, a small proportion of elderly patients never adapt, but remain in a perpetual 'Alice in Wonderland' world.

Contact lenses   Both hard and soft contact lenses may be used after cataract surgery. Following operation by the intracapsular method the corneal sensitivity is reduced, as a proportion of the corneal nerves have been cut. Discomfort is therefore not a problem, but difficulty with the handling of the lens or a general antipathy to the very idea of contact lenses sometimes make their use unsuitable.

The visual results are considerably better than with spectacles. The distortions are absent, as the lens moves with the cornea with any alteration of gaze. The magnifying effects are minimal so that the patient retains his normal-sized world.

Intraocular implants   The replacement of the diseased lens by a clear plastic lens is now becoming more popular with surgeons and patients.

The complications to the eye are gradually being reduced with improved microsurgical techniques. The lenses lie either in the anterior chamber or are suspended in or behind the pupil.

Problems in ophthalmology

They are inserted at the time of the removal of the cataract.

If there is contact between the lens and the corneal endothelium, either at the time of surgery or afterwards, the cells of the endothelium become damaged. As they are unable to regenerate like epithelial cells the cornea may become oedematous as aqueous leaks into it. When this major complication can be avoided, the results for the patient are dramatic. The distance vision is corrected and the patient can see as soon as the pad is removed postoperatively. For work he or she must use reading glasses like normal-sighted contemporaries.

The indications for the use of an intraocular lens are in the elderly patient who probably will not tolerate a contact lens or spectacles. The operation should not be carried out when there is only one functioning eye.

Chronic glaucoma

Introduction The fear of missing a case of chronic glaucoma is a worry for many doctors, resulting in the unnecessary referral of many patients. Unfortunately there is no easy way out of this dilemma and therefore, if in doubt, it is wise to refer patients for glaucoma screening.

Nature of the disease There is usually a rise in intraocular pressure above the normal level of 15–20 mmHg. This is probably due to a defect in the trabecular meshwork which lines the angle of the anterior chamber.

The raised intraocular pressure upsets the balance of the arterial perfusion pressure of the optic disc, resulting in the death of nerve tissue shown by cupping of the disc. This causes the characteristic losses in the field of vision.

Presentation This disease is insidious and the patient is usually unaware of any problems until the condition is well advanced.

Family history The condition rarely presents until after the age of 40 and there is often a family history of glaucoma.

Symptoms Pain in the eyes and headaches are very rare, unlike their presence in acute glaucoma.

Some difficulty with reading may suggest that a routine refraction for spectacles is necessary, when cupping of the disc is first noticed.

The normal disc The normal optic disc has a central depression – the physiological cup – and there is usually a marked similarity between the two eyes. The disc is pinker on the nasal than on the temporal side, and tends to be smaller with a less pronounced cup in hypermetropia or long sight.

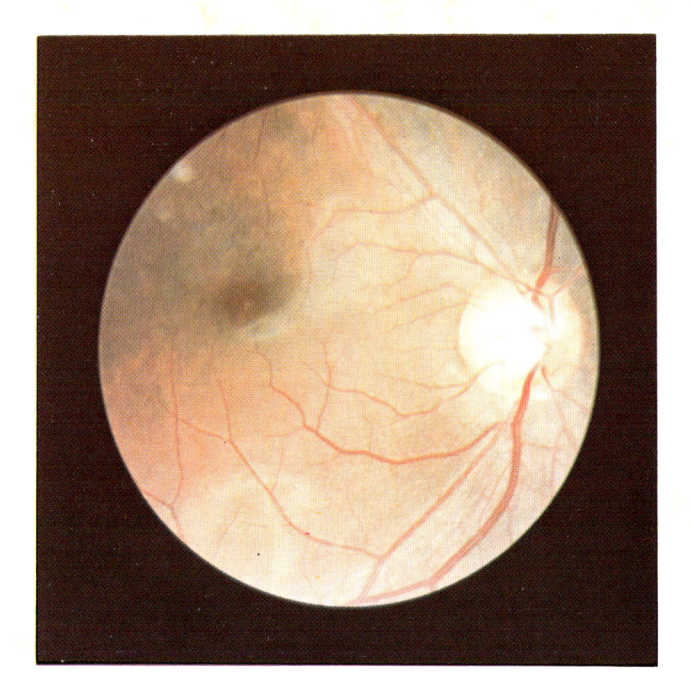

Figure 5.1   Normal fundus in a coloured person

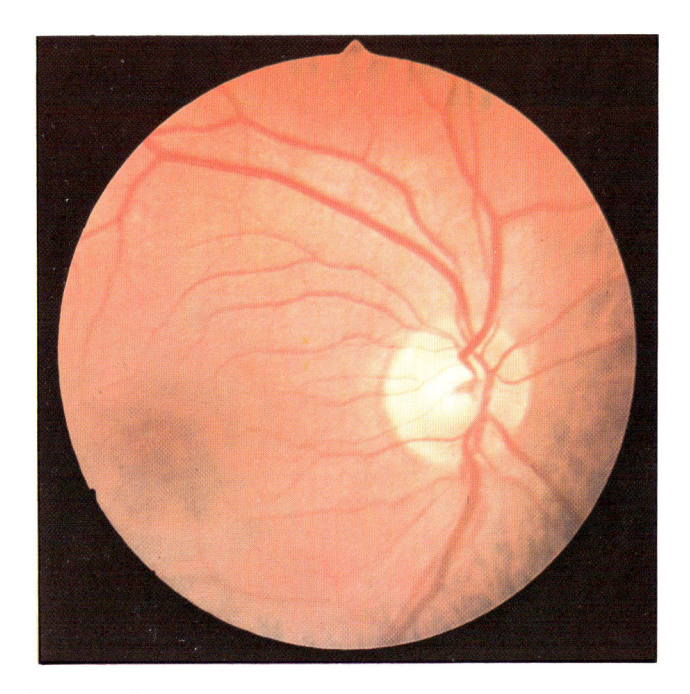

Figure 5.2   Normal fundus in a white person

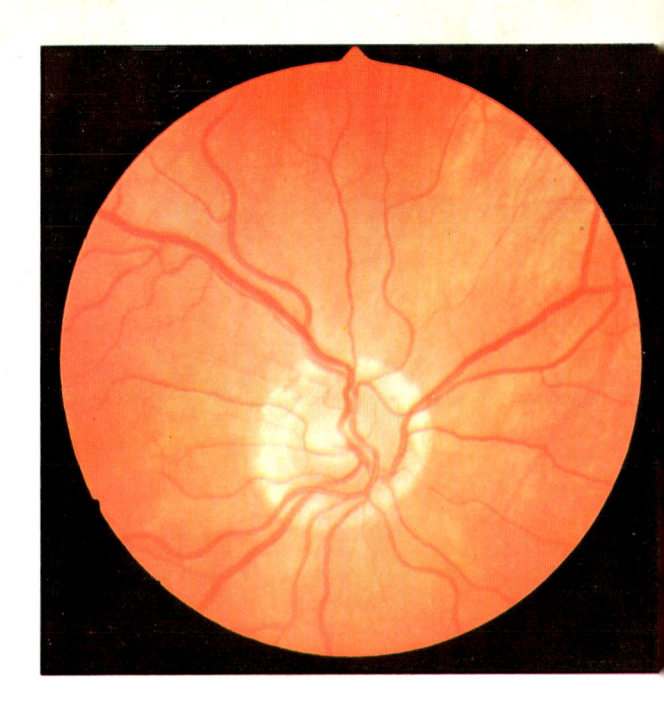

Figure 5.3 Normal disc showing 'halo' found in myopia

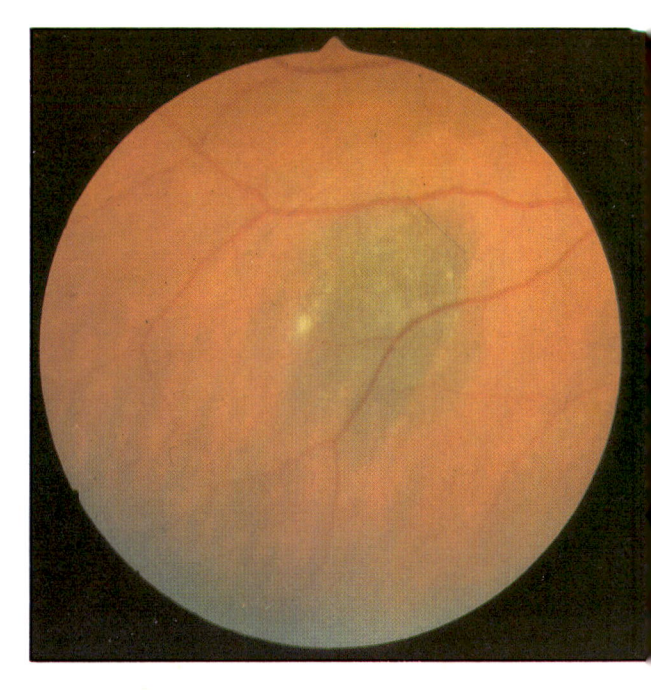

Figure 5.4 Choroidal naevus: a typical benign, flat, greyish lesion with feathery edges

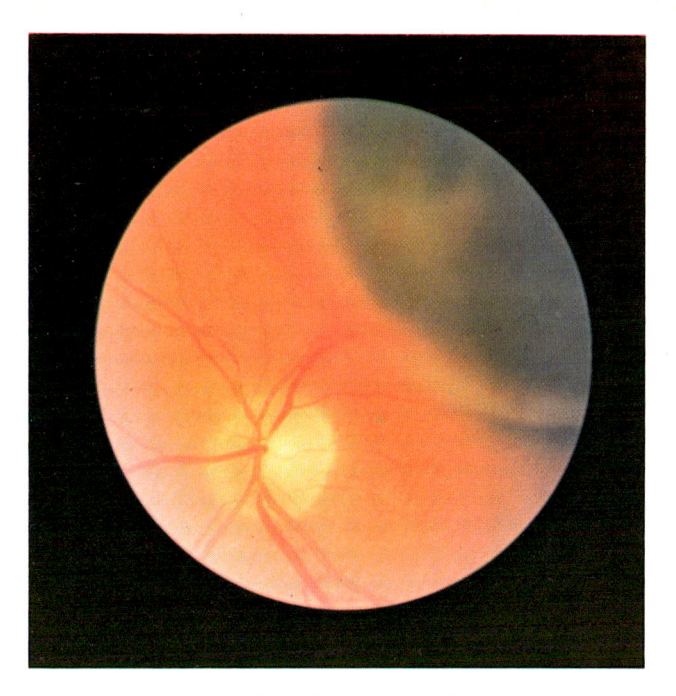

Figure 5.5 Choroidal malignant melanoma: a heavily pigmented tumour enlarging into the eye and metastazing most commonly to the liver

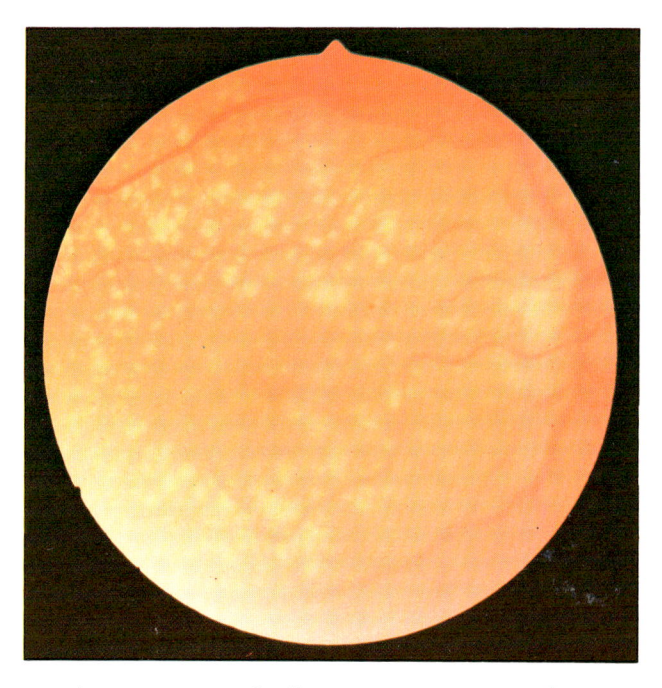

Figure 5.6 Drusen, appearing here as scattered yellow spots, may occur without any disturbance to central vision

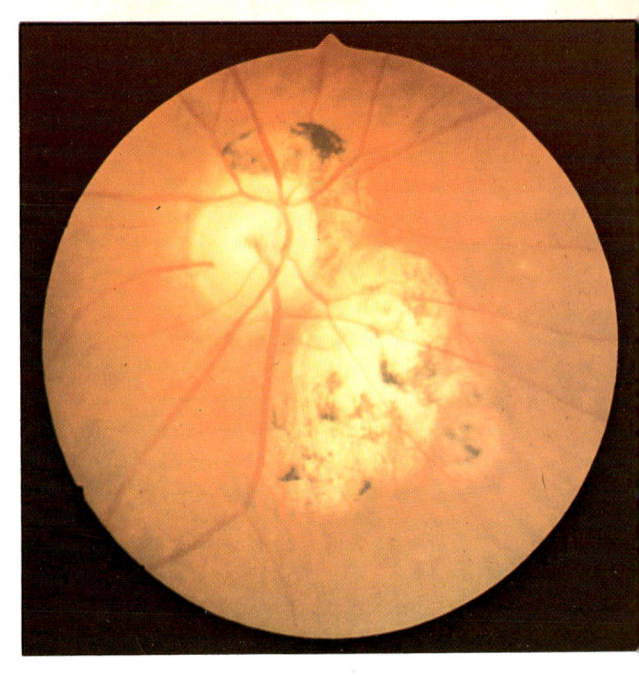

Figure 5.7 Toxoplasmosis: inactive lesions occurring next to the disc

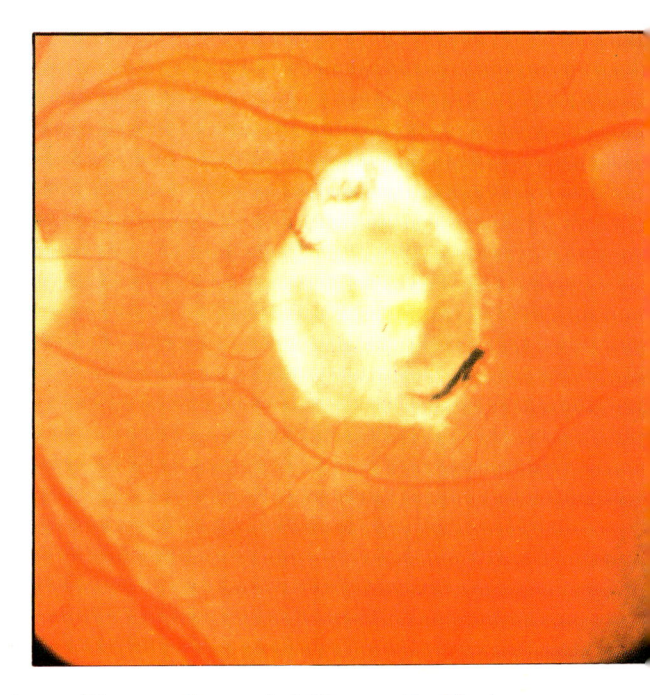

Figure 5.8 Toxocariasis: a white granuloma mimicking a retinoblastoma

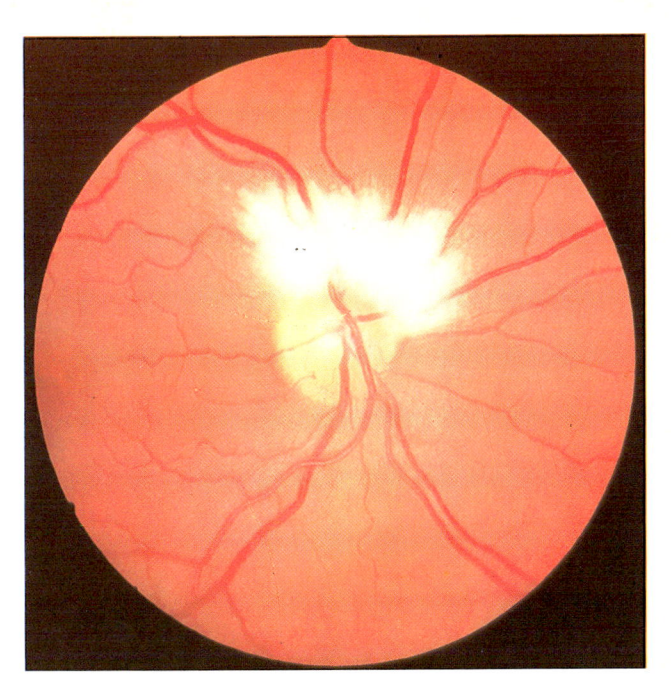

Figure 5.9 Medullation of retinal nerve fibres

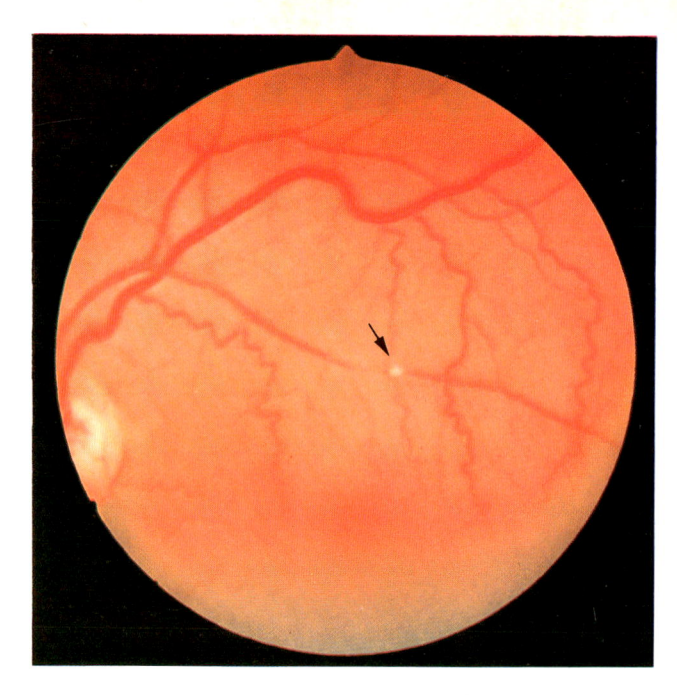

Figure 6.1 Cholesterol embolus (arrowed) from diseased carotid vessels causing transient loss of vision

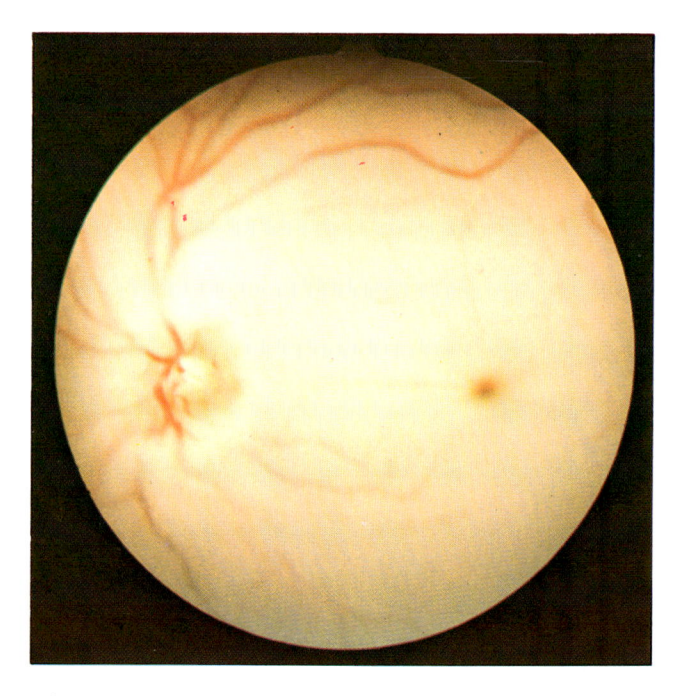

Figure 6.2 Central retinal artery occlusion: total loss of vision with white oedomatous retina, narrowed vessels and cherry-red macular spot

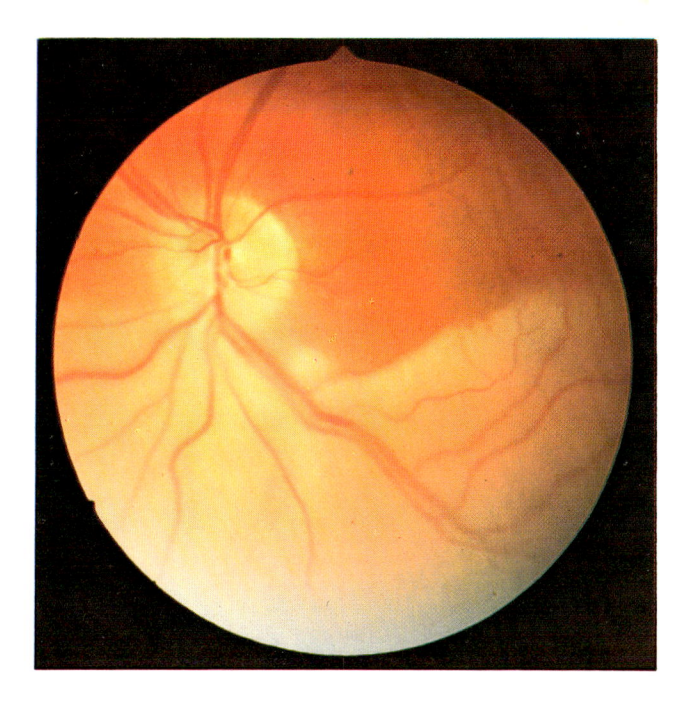

Figure 6.3 Branch retinal artery occlusion: oedema is limited to the lower half of the retina, causing an upper half defect in the visual field

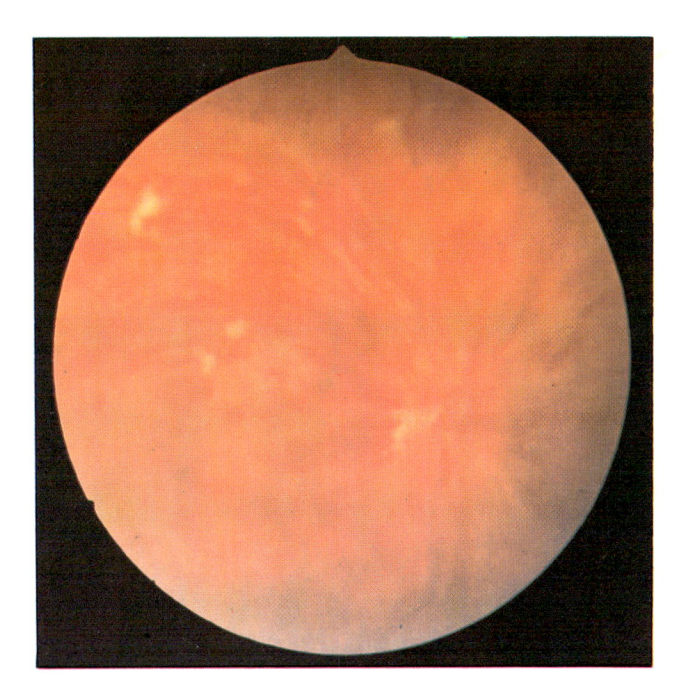

Figure 6.4 Central retinal vein occlusion: flame-shaped haemorrhages cover the retina and mask the disc

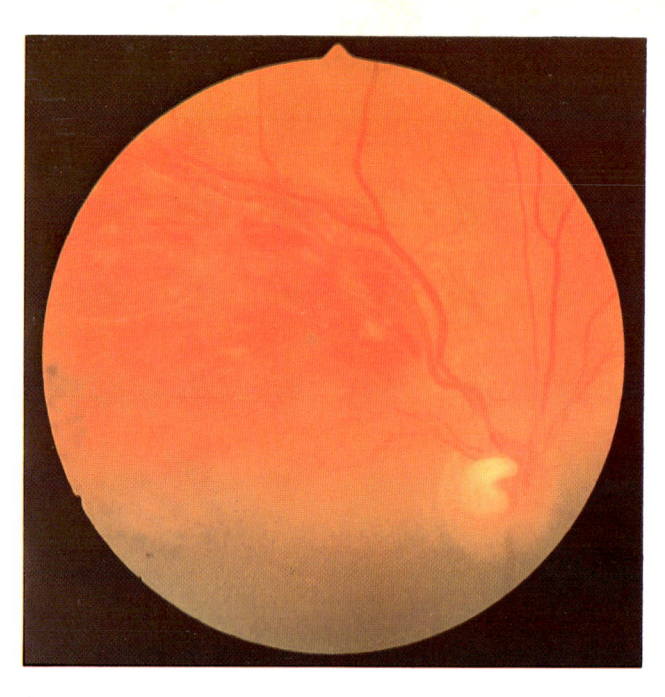

Figure 6.5 Branch retinal vein occlusion: there are retinal haemorrhages distal to the site of venous obstruction

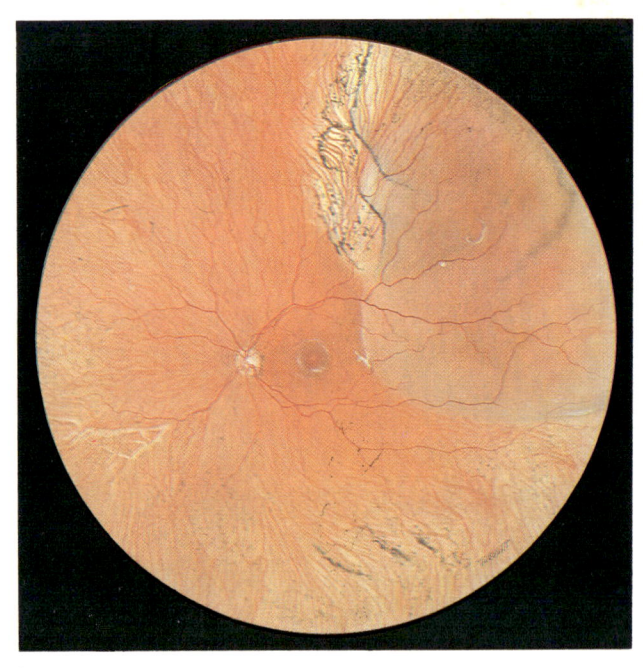

Figure 6.6 Retinal detachment: a raised grey area of retina extending from the periphery to the edge of the macula, with a single round tear

Slow loss of vision

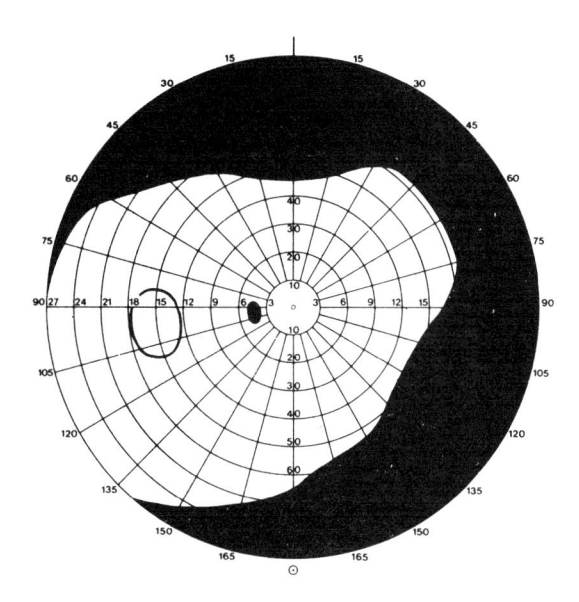

Normal left field of vision: peripheral and central field of left eye showing normal smaller nasal field due to the nose and the normal blind spot

Diagram 1

The cupped disc

The development of pathological changes is marked by a vertical enlargement of the cup to form an oval shape. The blood vessels dip over the edges of the notched upper and lower rims to reappear on the white atrophic base (**Figure 7.5**, p. 91).

Visual fields

Tests for the visual field changes in glaucoma are best left to a specialist. The confrontation method does not provide the detailed information about the central field of vision that is needed for the assessment for glaucoma.

The defects correspond with the changes seen at the optic disc. Extension of the cup inferiorly will produce a blind area (scotoma) in the upper half of the visual field. This becomes continuous (arcuate scotoma) with the normal blind spot which is also enlarged (Diagrams 1 & 2). The arcuate defects gradually link with the loss in either the upper or lower nasal field (Diagram 3). There is an inevitable progression in the untreated case, but the central vision is retained until a very late stage (Diagram 4). This is the reason why some patients are unaware of the extent of their condition as they have normal visual acuity and can read.

Problems in ophthalmology

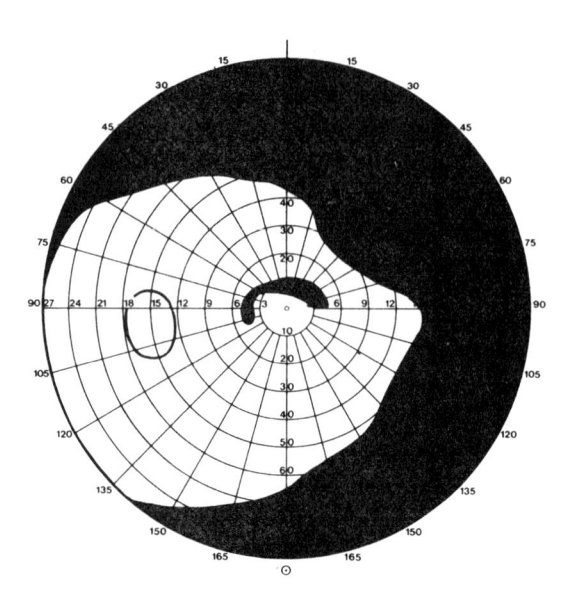

Glaucomatous field defects: an area of visual loss extending from the blind spot (arcuate scotoma), and loss of the upper nasal field (nasal step)

Diagram 2

Intraocular pressure

The digital method for measuring intraocular pressure has no place in the assessment for chronic glaucoma. Referral for testing by applanation tonometry or the recently-introduced air tonometry method is obligatory.

Occasionally the intraocular pressure may appear within normal limits despite obvious cupping of the disc. This is then classified as 'low tension' glaucoma and is managed in the same way as chronic glaucoma.

The opposite finding is raised intraocular pressure in the absence of any field defect. This is ocular hypertension and may precede chronic glaucoma. Patients with this condition must then be kept under review.

Association with systemic disease

Chronic glaucoma is three times more likely to occur in diabetic than non-diabetic patients. Diabetic patients who have the condition also tend to develop visual field defects more easily.

Hypertensive patients, especially those who are diabetic, with chronic glaucoma are also at risk if the blood pressure is lowered suddenly by an alteration of their drug therapy.

Slow loss of vision

Diagram 3

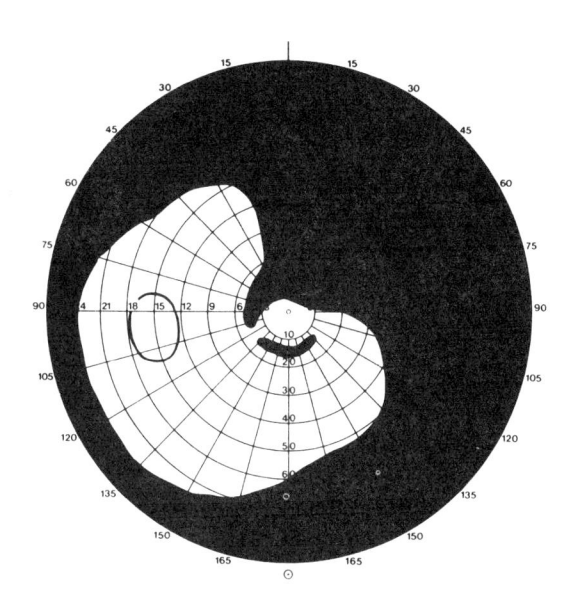

Glaucomatous field defects: the upper arcuate scotoma has linked with the nasal step. A lower arcuate scotoma has appeared

Presumably poor arterial perfusion of the optic disc produces the marked increase in field defects.

Management

The control of all cases of chronic glaucoma should be by an eye department.

Three criteria are used to estimate the success of treatment: charting of the field of vision, measurement of intraocular pressure and the appearance of the discs.

Many sophisticated field charting devices are being produced in an attempt to standardize the results. It is doubtful however – in view of the considerable expense of these computerized machines – that their use can be justified other than as research tools.

Non-contact tonometers can record the intraocular pressures without touching the eye. This method is now commonly used when patients are refracted for spectacles. While detecting a few early cases of glaucoma, the method also produces a considerable number of false positives, particularly when used by inexperienced hands. All these cases, however, should be referred for a full glaucoma screening.

Problems in ophthalmology

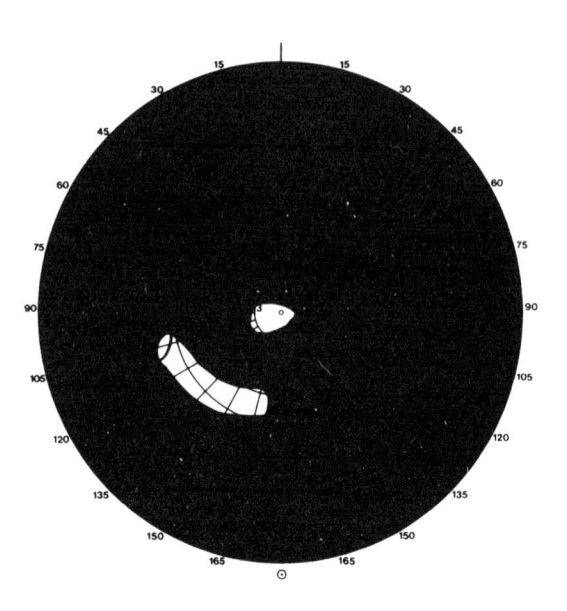

Glaucomatous field defects: loss of all the field of vision except for two small areas in an untreated case of chronic simple glaucoma

Diagram 4

Changes in the appearance of the disc in glaucoma can be recorded numerically. The ratio of the diameter of the cup to the diameter of the disc is estimated (cup/disc ratio or C/D ratio). When the cup is half the diameter of the disc the C/D ratio is 0.5. If the cupping is extensive it may increase to 0.9 when almost the entire disc is cupped.

In general it should be explained to all patients that their condition is chronic, requiring assessment for the remainder of their lives, that the visual field defects cannot be reversed as they are due to death of nerve tissue, and that successful treatment will have been achieved if further deterioration is prevented. This is a rather negative approach for a patient who often feels that after careful use of his drops there should be some improvement in his vision. It must be stressed to the patient that if treatment is stopped the intraocular pressure will rise and further loss of vision will occur.

Rather as with the recently diagnosed diabetic, the initial keenness of the new glaucoma patient to comply with the doctor's orders tends to lapse with the passing years. Occasion-

Slow loss of vision

ally the use of drops becomes haphazard despite the protestations and denials from the patient and the intraocular pressure is found to be raised. It may be necessary to admit the patient for 48 hours in order to assess the pressure when the treatment has been given regularly. This method of 'phasing' is also used when the visual field defects increase in the presence of apparently normal intraocular pressure. It is then often found that the control of the pressure is not maintained throughout the 24 hours and that at some time it is raised, necessitating an alteration in the treatment.

Medical treatment

Medical treatment for chronic glaucoma consists of local application of drops and systemic carbonic anhydrase inhibitors.

Local treatment
Pilocarpine

Pilocarpine drops are the most widely prescribed treatment. It is given in strengths of 1–4% every 6 hours each day as it has an effective action for up to 6 hours.

The cholinergic action of the drug causes constriction of the pupil and contraction of the ciliary muscle. The miosis of the

Side-effects

pupil causes some dimming of the vision. This may be particularly marked in patients with central cataracts in whom the drug may produce considerable visual deterioration which lasts as long as the pupil is constricted.

In the younger patient, the effect on the ciliary muscle alters the focus of the lens so that the eye becomes myopic. This blurring of vision lasts for about 1 hour and may be severe enough to prevent the continued use of the drug.

Mild discomfort or occasionally pain may be felt in the eye for the first few days, but this generally becomes tolerable.

Adrenaline

Adrenaline drops either 0.5% or 1% have an adrenergic effect on the eye and are given twice daily.

Side-effects

The pupillary dilation that also occurs restricts the use of adrenaline to cases in which the angle is open. If the anterior chamber is shallow there is a risk of precipitating angle closure or acute glaucoma.

Adrenaline tends to cause discomfort when instilled and may produce redness.

Guanethidine

Guanethidine may be given with adrenaline whose action it enhances. A gritty discomfort and redness of the eye may limit its use.

Timoptol

The adrenergic drug timoptol is the latest addition to the treatment of glaucoma. It is given as 0.25% or 0.5% drops twice daily and is free of the unpleasant side-effects of both pilo-

Problems in ophthalmology

carpine and adrenaline. Unfortunately, the cost is high.

Side-effects   Timoptol must be used with caution in patients with asthma, bradycardia or heart failure as it may be absorbed.

Systemic treatment   Carbonic anhydrase inhibitors, acetazolamide (Diamox) and dichlorphenamide (Daranide or Oratrol) may be used to supplement the action of local treatment. Both work by reducing the secretion of aqueous.

Side-effects   Unpleasant side-effects are common, with paraesthesia in the hands and feet, indigestion and loss of appetite. Occasionally patients may become depressed and lose weight and the risk of these compounds contributing to formation of renal calculi can limit their use in anyone with kidney disease.

Surgical treatment

Surgical treatment is only considered if medical treatment has failed to control the condition. This may occur because the pressure remains too high despite treatment or because of poor compliance by the patient due to unpleasant side-effects or simply his or her failing to use the treatment on a regular basis.

Drainage operations   Numerous methods have been devised to help the drainage of aqueous from the eye, but the method most commonly used at the present time is trabeculectomy.

The operation is performed under local or general anaesthesia with a hospital stay of about 1 week. Return to sedentary work is possible within 1 month. The operation may alter the focus of the eye so that a change in spectacle correction may be necessary.

Macular degeneration

Introduction   Senile macular degeneration is the commonest cause of blindness in the United Kingdom, but while the condition is progressive and untreatable there is much advice and help that can be given to patients.

Presentation   The patient tends to notice a gradual deterioration of his or her vision. At first straight lines may develop a kink due to the separation by oedema of the cone receptor cells at the macula. Objects may appear smaller than usual (micropsia) and the normal colour values are changed.

These early symptoms are replaced by a central haze or greyness and eventually by a total blind area in the central field of vision.

The patient may attempt to overcome the problem by

Slow loss of vision

looking slightly to one side of an object or to scan across it in order to use normal adjacent retinal cones. By this method a level of 6/36 or even 6/24 can sometimes be achieved. Unfortunately the near vision is not proportionately as good and reading becomes impossible. Occasionally the loss may be sudden when a haemorrhage develops and blots out all useful central vision.

Clinical findings
As macular degeneration is an ageing change it may be difficult to examine the fundi because of senile miosis and cataract. It is then necessary to dilate the pupils to achieve a satisfactory view of the retina.

In the early stages there is a distortion of the normal foveal reflex. Clumping of black or grey pigment is seen around the fovea (**Figure 7.6**, p. 92).

The degree of visual failure does not always equate with the changes seen at the macula. Marked visual loss may occur with minimal ophthalmoscopic change or alternatively it is sometimes difficult to know how a patient can see with such an apparently abnormal macula.

Disciform degeneration
A rather more dramatic appearance occurs with disciform degeneration of the macula. Initially the macula appears grey and elevated due to a choroidal haemorrhage beneath the retina. Sometimes the haemorrhage breaks through into the retina and is seen around the edge of the grey area. Over a period of months the elevated area turns white due to scarring and the central vision is finally lost (**Figure 7.7**, p. 92).

Management
While there is no treatment that will prevent the progression of macular degeneration there is much supportive help that the general practitioner can give.

Explanation of the condition
The patient often seeks attention, thinking that all that is needed is a change of spectacles, only to be told by his optician that the prescription is correct. The nature of the condition can best be explained to the patient by comparing the eye with a camera. When the camera lens has been focussed correctly, it is then necessary to have an undamaged film to record the picture. Any dust or spots on the film will prevent this.

In the eye, damage to the macular area of the retina results in central loss of vision.

Low visual aids
The vision may be helped by enlarging the image so that it falls on a greater number of retinal cones. This can most easily be done with a magnifying glass. The lens may be held in the hand or may be mounted on various types of stand.

Similar magnification can be achieved with stronger reading glasses, but the working distance may be so short that it is impracticable.

A telescopic low visual aid may be added to the spectacles so that only one eye is used. The device is like half a pair of opera glasses. It may be adjusted for distance viewing or for reading by changing one of the lenses mounted on the front. The increased magnification is accompanied by a decreased visual field so that they cannot be worn for walking around.

Correct lighting will often improve the performance of a failing macula and some low visual aids incorporate a light, similar to an illuminated magnifying glass for map reading.

These low visual aids when used correctly may help to preserve a sense of independence in a patient with failing vision. The ability to sign a cheque, look up a telephone number or even trim one's finger nails is accepted by the normal sighted and it is only when this ability is lost that we realize how much we take for granted in our visually-dependent world.

Senile macular degeneration is usually a bilateral condition although one eye may be involved earlier. In such a case the patient may prefer to shut the affected eye and so prevent the central blur from being superimposed on the clear retinal image of the normal eye. This should be encouraged and the patient reassured that no extra strain is thrown on the normal eye.

Many patients admit that they limit their reading to try to save their failing vision. Unfortunately the degenerative process is not related to use, so that the patient should be told to use the eyes as normally as the level of vision permits.

With the inevitable progression of the disease, albeit sometimes over several years, the doctor must be in a position to offer something positive. It certainly helps the patient to know that the condition only affects the central vision. Regardless of how bad the central vision becomes, the peripheral vision will remain normal. This side vision is essential as 'navigational vision' to prevent knocking into furniture in a room or into people in a crowded street.

Registration as partially sighted or blind

When the visual acuity has fallen to less than 6/18, depending on any peripheral visual field loss it may be possible to register the patient. This should be carried out after examination by an ophthalmologist and will result in the patient being placed on either the partially sighted or the blind register. This registration is important because of the benefits it may confer (Table 7.1).

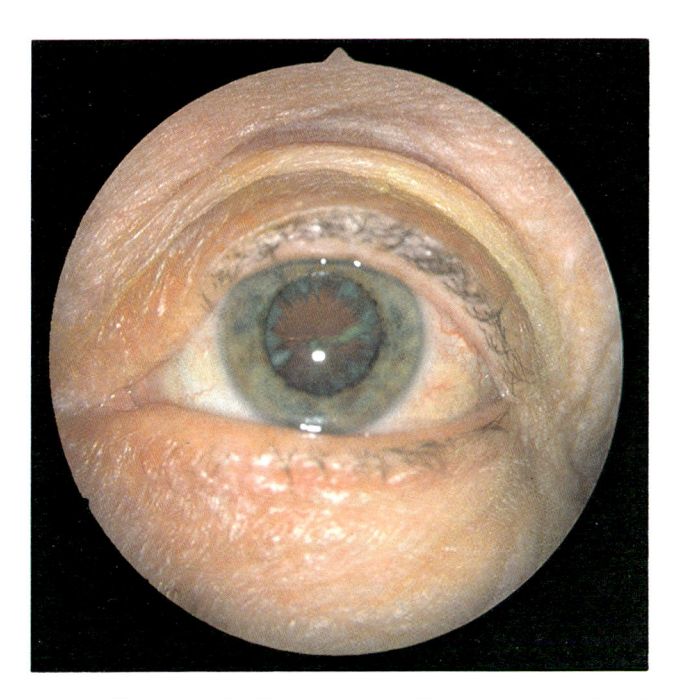

Figure 7.1 Cortical cataract: radiating spoke-like opacities affecting the peripheral lens with a few extensions towards the centre. Visual acuity may be good until central opacities develop

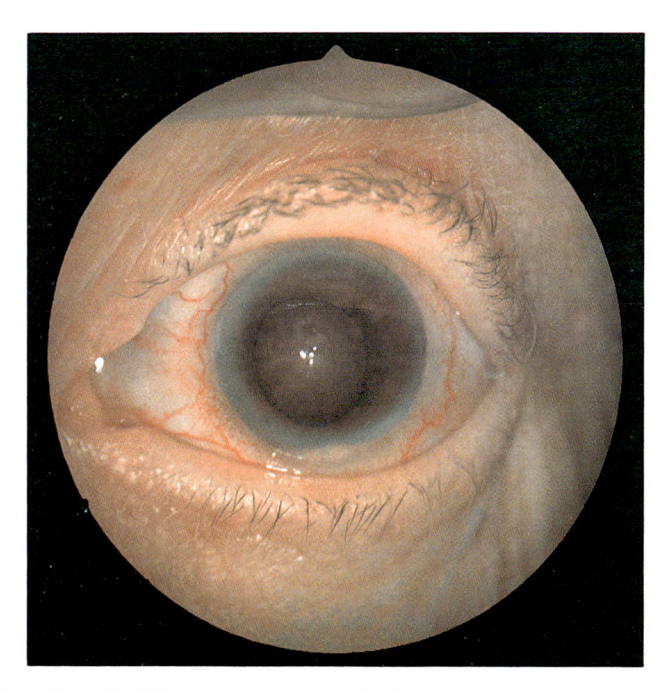

Figure 7.2 Nuclear sclerosis: a dark brown cataract in the late stages

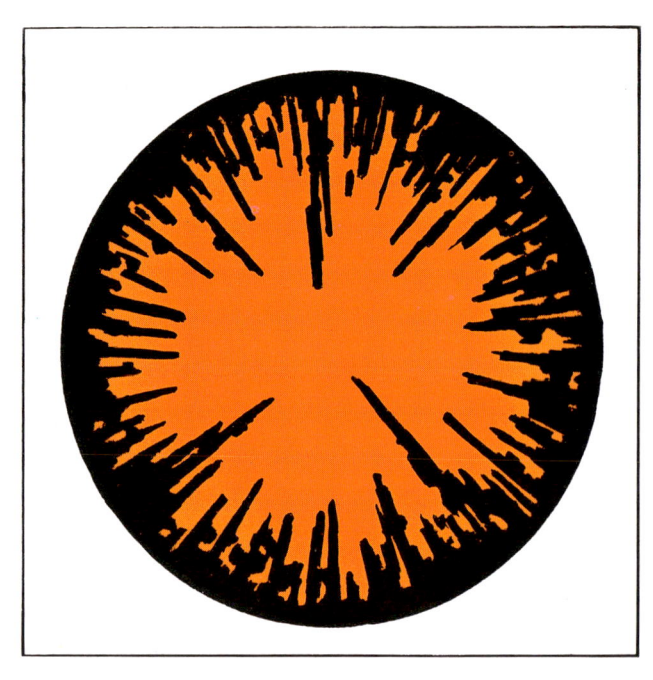

Figure 7.3 Cortical cataract: silhouette of spoke opacities

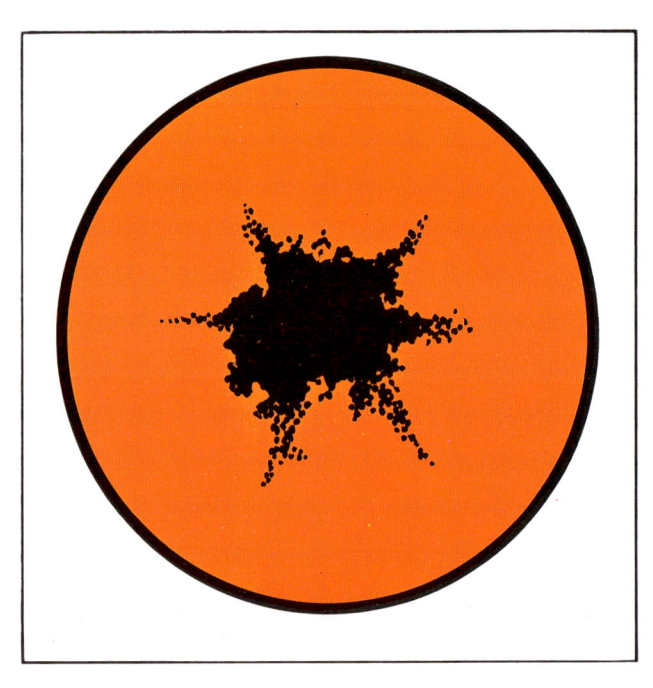

Figure 7.4 Cortical cataract: silhouette of posterior subcapsular opacities

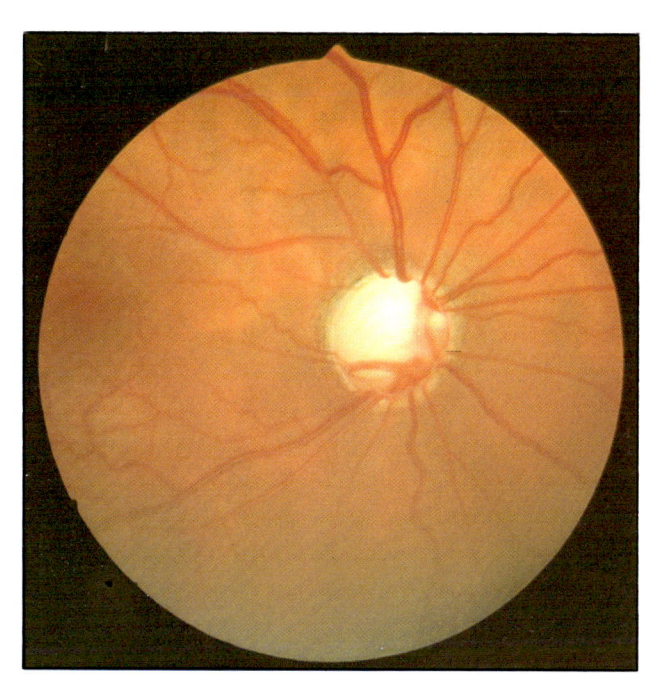

Figure 7.5 Disc cupping: advanced case with the vessels disappearing over the edge of the cupped disc

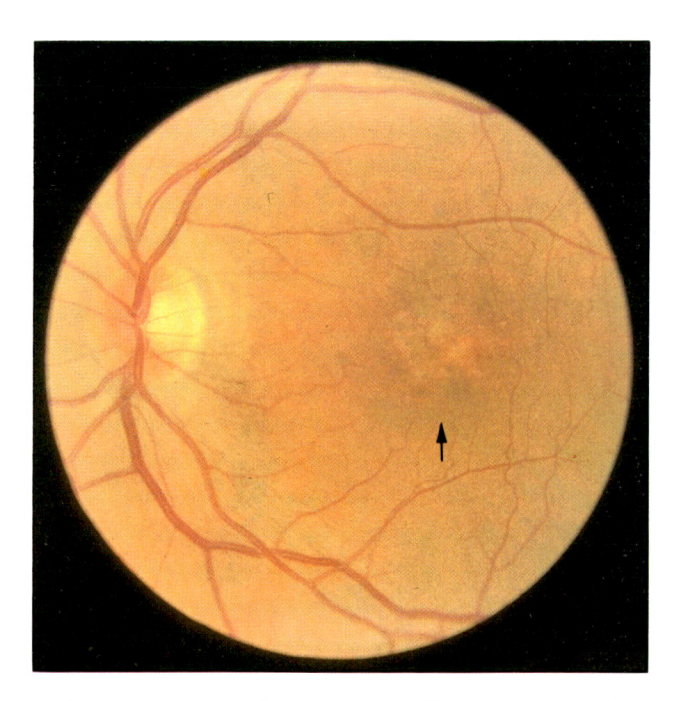

Figure 7.6 Senile macular degeneration: patchy pigmentary change occurs only at the macula

Figure 7.7 Disciform degeneration of the macula, showing an organized white scar, formation of which renders the loss of central vision irreversible

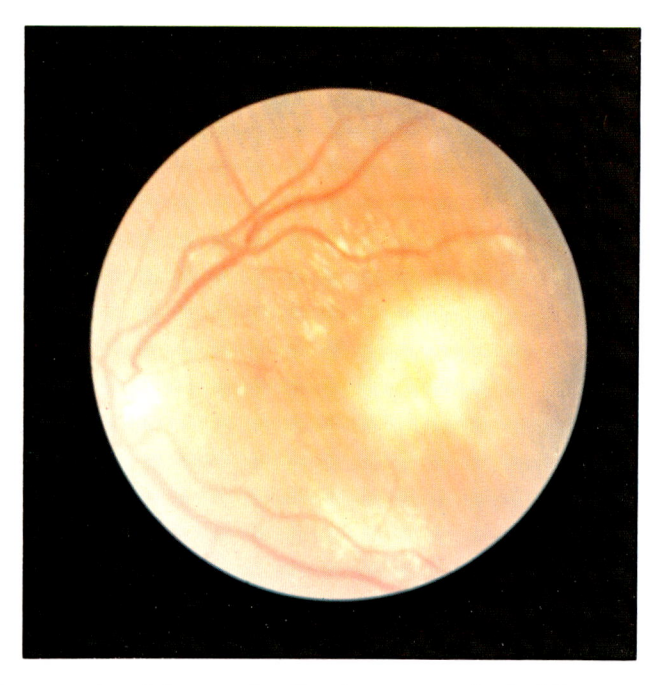

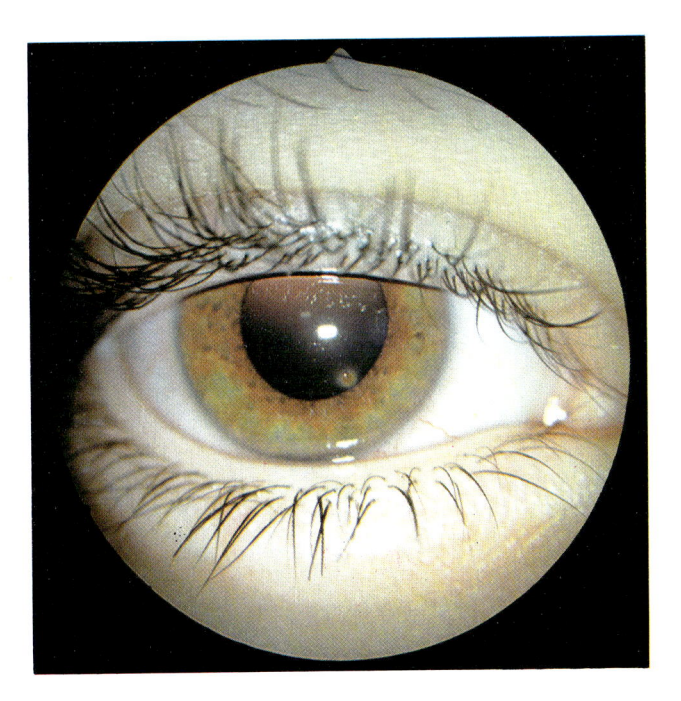

Figure 8.1 Corneal foreign body

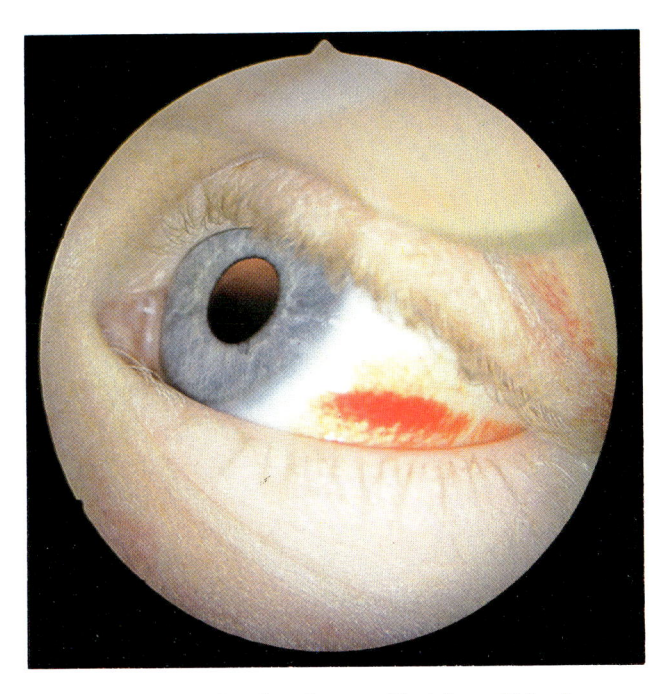

Figure 8.2 Subconjunctival haemorrhage: localized area of bright-red blood

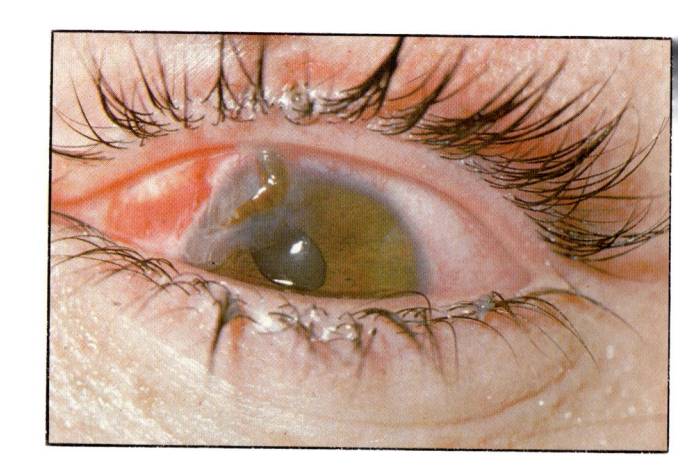

Figure 8.3 Corneal laceration: full thickness laceration with iris prolapse. The pupil is oval-shaped and drawn towards the wound

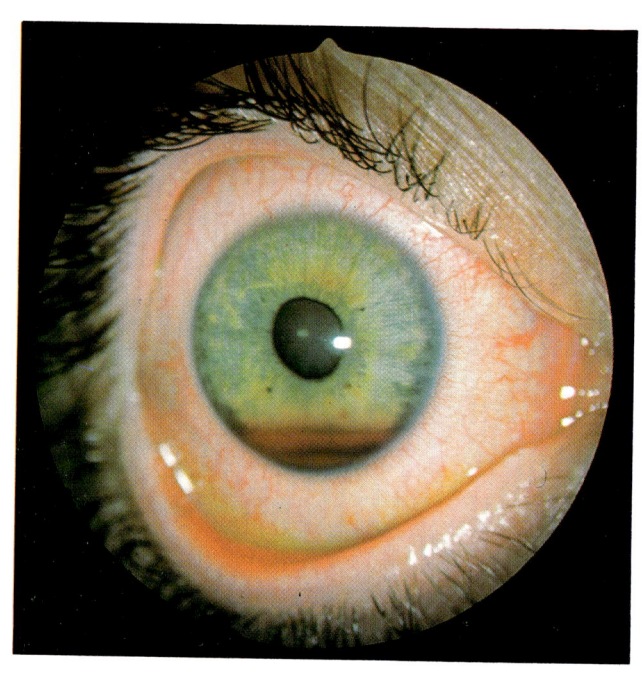

Figure 8.4 Hyphaema: blood level in the lower half of the anterior chamber

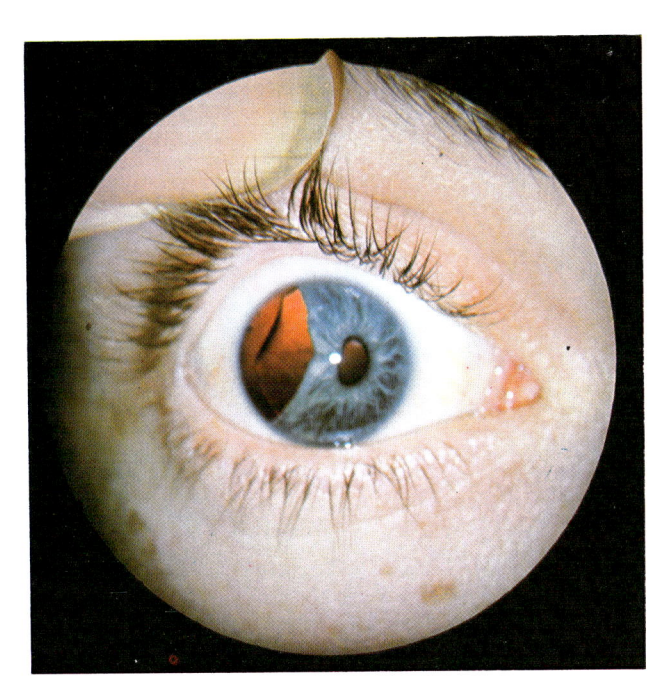

Figure 8.5 Iridodyalisis: the root of the iris has been torn by .22 airgun pellet, causing double vision

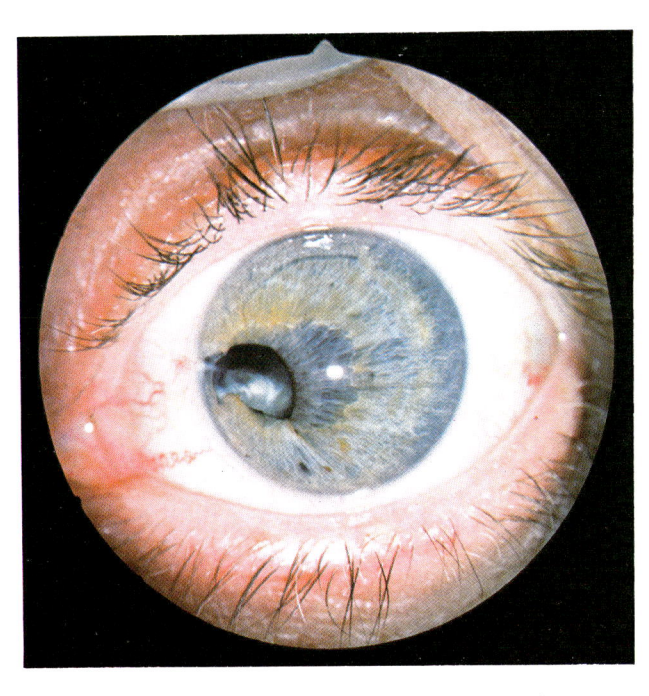

Figure 8.6 Cataract: a penetrating injury at the limbus has resulted in displacement of the pupil towards the wound and a localized opacity in the lens

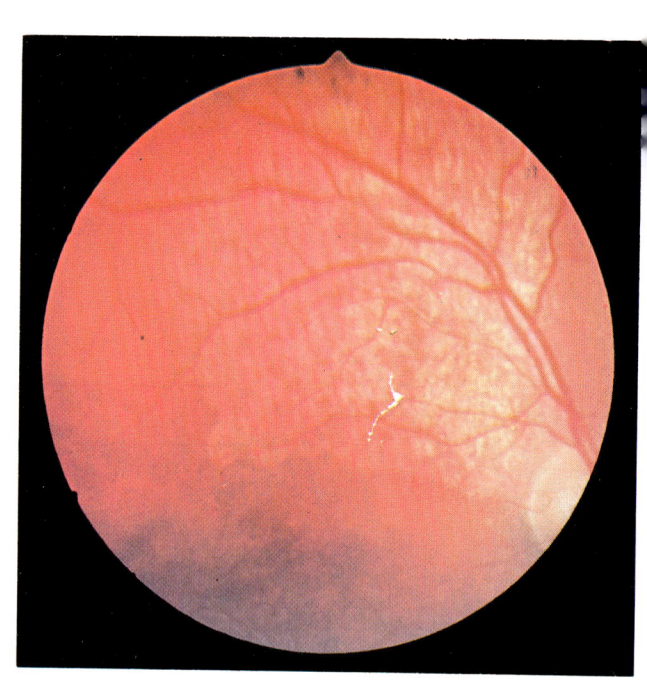

Figure 8.7 Commotio retinae: white retinal oedema caused by a blow from a football

Slow loss of vision

Table 7.1

Partially sighted register benefits

Talking book service
Visiting service
Holidays
White stick

Blind register benefits

Financial help on supplementary allowance
Free radio
Talking book service
Holidays
Income tax relief
Television licence reduction
Guide dog
Various aids
   disabled badge for car
   household equipment

8 Trauma

Introduction – Superficial injuries – Lacerations – Penetrating injuries – Blunt injury – Chemical injuries – Radiation injuries

Introduction

All eye injuries, with the exception of the most superficial, require specialist treatment. However, while the obvious cases demand no great diagnostic skill, hidden damage can occur to the ocular structures, making careful examination essential if the injury is not to be overlooked.

Superficial injuries

Symptoms | There is extreme pain and profuse watering of the eye. The marked protective spasm of the lids, which may prevent adequate examination, may be relieved by instilling a short-acting local anaesthetic (oxybuprocaine (Minims Benoxinate)).

Babies should be wrapped in a blanket and laid on a couch. An assistant, preferably not the parent, should hold the head and pull down the lower lid of the affected eye, while the examiner lifts the upper lid.

Corneal foreign bodies Removal | Foreign bodies on the cornea may be brushed off with a cotton-wool bud or may require removal with a sterile hypodermic needle. If a needle is used, it is more easily held if attached to a syringe.

Local antibiotic ointment is instilled and the eye is firmly padded.

Mydriasis | Any break in the epithelium usually heals within 24 hours. Mydriatic drops are only needed if the eye remains inflamed, in

Problems in ophthalmology

which case a short-acting drug is given (homatropine or cyclopentolate). *Never* use atropine.

Rust rings
If a rust ring remains after removal of a corneal foreign body, local antibiotic should be instilled, the eye padded and the patient referred that day to an eye department (**Figure 8.1**, p. 93).

Subtarsal foreign bodies
If no corneal foreign body is found, the upper lid should be everted. Subtarsal foreign bodies tend to lodge just behind the lid margin. If nothing is found, it is useful to wipe the inside of the lid with cotton wool. This may remove any foreign body that is the same colour as the lid and difficult to see.

Corneal abrasion
The symptoms of corneal abrasion are similar to those of a foreign body.

Cause
The corneal epithelium may be damaged as a result of a wide range of injuries. Amongst the commonest are mishandling of contact lenses, or hitting of the eye by a finger nail or a twig.

Findings
Fluorescein dye will stain the affected area and differentiate the condition from an overlooked subtarsal foreign body.

Treatment
Local antibiotic ointment is given and the eye firmly padded until the abrasion has healed.

Recurrent erosion
The patient complains of repeated attacks of waking with a painful watering eye that settles within a few hours.

Cause
The condition is due to a breakdown of the corneal epithelium, usually at the site of a previous abrasion.

Unless the patient is seen when the eye is painful no corneal staining is elicited with fluorescein dye.

The condition is diagnosed by the typical history of recurrent attacks.

Treatment
The acute abrasion is treated with antibiotic ointment and padding. Thereafter, continued use of ointment at night for 6–8 weeks may be helpful.

Lacerations

Skin
Cuts around the eyes tend to bleed profusely, which may mask injury to the globe. However, the vascularity means that wounds heal well.

Lacerations involving the lid margin must be sutured with accuracy to avoid notching of the margin or trichiasis. Débridement should be avoided unless there is such obvious damage to tissue that it is not viable.

Especial caution should be taken when the medial ends of the lids are involved, as the lachrymal ducts may be damaged. Lacerations of the lower canaliculus must be repaired under the

Trauma

microscope using a splint of polythene tubing inserted into the cut ends of the duct to prevent scarring and narrowing.

Conjunctiva — Lacerations of the conjunctiva alone are not serious and require no treatment unless extensive. However, there may be damage to the underlying sclera.

Subconjunctival haemorrhage takes up to 2 weeks to absorb during which time it retains the bright red appearance (**Figure 8.2**, p. 93).

Penetrating injuries

Cornea and sclera — Rupture of the cornea or sclera allows not only the loss of intraocular contents, but also an easy access for infection.

Small wounds of the cornea may be self-sealing and require only padding.

When there is dark-coloured tissue extruding from a corneal or scleral wound the uveal tract is involved (**Figure 8.3**, p. 94). Depending on the severity of the injury, the pupil may be distorted towards the wound, the anterior chamber may be absent, or the whole globe may be collapsed if vitreous has been lost.

In all cases the eye should be covered with a sterile swab and lightly bandaged. No local drops or ointment should be instilled. Immediate referral is indicated for examination and repair, if necessary under a general anaesthetic.

X-ray for intraocular foreign body — The eye should always be X-rayed if there is a history of hammering or drilling, to exclude an intraocular foreign body. The entry wound in these cases may be minute and easily missed. While some substances (glass and plastic) are inert, copper and iron foreign bodies disintegrate if left in the eye. The metal becomes deposited in all the tissues and results in a sterile endophthalmitis and blindness.

Blunt injury

Non-penetrating injuries may cause immediate symptoms with blurred or total loss of vision. Alternatively the effects may not appear until long after the acute episode has subsided.

Haematoma — The tissues of the lids are easily distensible so that even minor trauma can result in considerable swelling. However, the common occurrence of the typical 'black eye' should not exclude a proper examination.

Examination — The vision should be checked, if the lids can be opened, and the brightness of the cornea assessed. The depth of the anterior chamber and the presence of any blood should be noted.

Problems in ophthalmology

Blow-out fracture

The movements of the eyes should be compared to see if there is any limitation of elevation of the affected eye, suggesting a blow-out fracture.

This injury is typically caused by a blow from a fist. The eye appears sunken and its upward movement is restricted due to the trapping of the inferior eye muscles in the fractured orbital floor. The patient should be referred to an eye department as surgical intervention may be indicated. Usually an operation does not prove necessary and full recovery occurs spontaneously.

Anterior chamber hyphaema

Bleeding from torn iris vessels causes a hyphaema. This may vary in size from a small collection of blood forming a level in the lower half of the anterior chamber (**Figure 8.4**, p. 94) to a total obscuration of the iris.

Management

All patients should be referred for admission. Although the blood absorbs within a few days, there is always a risk of secondary bleeding occurring between the third and fifth days. When the anterior chamber has cleared, the pupil may be dilated safely so that a detailed examination of the fundus is possible.

Occasionally a complete hyphaema which fills the anterior chamber also obstructs the angle, causing glaucoma. The blood must be evacuated to relieve the glaucoma and prevent staining of the cornea by haemosiderin.

Iris

Tears of the root of the iris producing iridodialysis are uncommon (**Figure 8.5**, p. 95). They may cause double vision, due to the extra 'pupil' that is formed, and require surgery. More commonly the iris sphincter muscle is damaged with the result that the pupil remains permanently dilated (traumatic mydriasis).

Lens

The lens may become dislocated resulting in distortion of the vision. Rupture of some of the fibres of the suspensory ligament allows the lens to move to one side. Rarely the lens may be dislocated backwards into the vitreous.

In all cases patients should be referred to an eye clinic so that a full assessment can be made.

Cataract formation is usually a late complication of non-penetrating injury. Either all or part of the lens becomes opaque and cataract extraction may be necessary (**Figure 8.6**, p. 95).

Retina

Haemorrhage from the retina into the vitreous causes marked reduction in vision.

Haemorrhage

The red reflex is absent even after the usual accompanying hyphaema has absorbed.

The patient must be admitted to hospital for complete bed

Trauma

Oedema

rest and to allow a detailed examination of the retina.

Oedema of the retina (commotio retinae) appears glistening-white and settles within one week (**Figure 8.7**, p. 96). It may be replaced by patchy pigmentary change which is serious when the macula is involved.

Detachment

Tears may occur in the thin peripheral retina that is found in myopic eyes and cause a retinal detachment.

Retinal tears or retinal dialysis may occur in normal eyes when the extreme periphery of the retina becomes torn. In all cases the retinal detachment may not become apparent for weeks or even months after the original injury and even then only when the macula is involved and the central vision lost.

All cases must be referred immediately for surgical treatment.

Chemical injuries

Chemical injuries to the eyes require instant action. The efficiency of the first-aid treatment will determine the eventual visual outcome.

Immediate irrigation with water

There is no time to identify the agent, ponder its toxicology or even obtain the appropriate antidote.

The eye must be irrigated immediately with large volumes of water. Local anaesthetic drops will help to overcome the inevitable blepharospasm.

If there are any particles of chemical, especially lime, these should be removed and care should be taken to examine the upper fornix when the upper lid has been everted.

Only when the eye has been adequately irrigated should it be padded and the patient transferred to an eye hospital.

Acid versus alkali

Acid burns tend to be self-limiting due to coagulation of protein. This is in contrast to the damage produced by alkalis such as lime or ammonia, which penetrate the eye rapidly causing marked iritis and cataract formation.

The long-term management of chemical burns is complicated, with treatment aimed at preventing the lids adhering to the globe (symblepharon) and limiting the intraocular inflammatory response.

Radiation injuries

Damage to the eye depends on the penetration of the ocular tissues by radiation of differing wavelengths.

Problems in ophthalmology

Ultraviolet radiation

Arc eye and snow blindness

Ultraviolet radiation injuries occur most commonly from misuse of sunray lamps, welding equipment (arc eye) or occasionally from reflected sunlight (snow blindness).

Ultraviolet light is largely absorbed by the cornea and conjunctiva and produces its effects by conjunctival hyperaemia and the loss of superficial epithelial cells of the cornea.

The symptoms do not start until several hours after exposure. Then there is intense photophobia, watering and grittiness.

Antibiotic ointment should be instilled and the eyes firmly padded. Analgesics may be needed to overcome the acute discomfort, which usually subsides within 24 hours. Local anaesthetic agents should not be used as they delay epithelial healing.

Infrared radiation

Eclipse burn

Infrared radiation is uncommon. Burns of the macula can occur while watching an eclipse of the sun – eclipse burn.

There is immediate variable loss of the central vision with a small discrete patch of pigmentary change in identical positions in the two eyes. As no treatment is possible, prevention is of paramount importance. The sun should never be viewed, even through a dense filter. An image of an eclipse can be obtained by making a pinhole in a piece of card and projecting the light onto black paper.

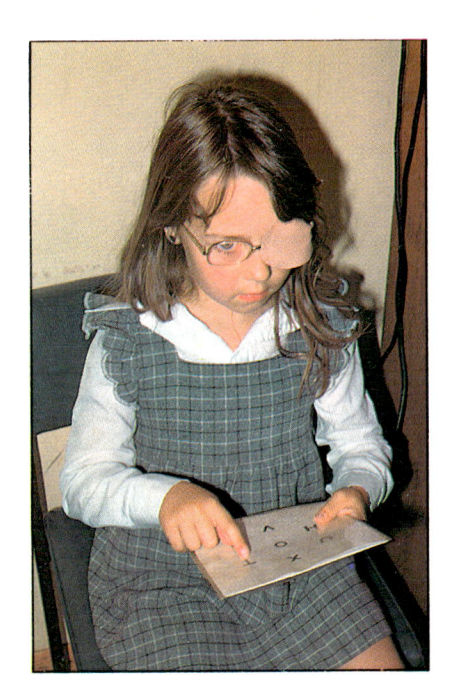

Figure 9.1 Sheridan Gardiner Test. This is used to test visual acuity in the 3–5-year-old age group

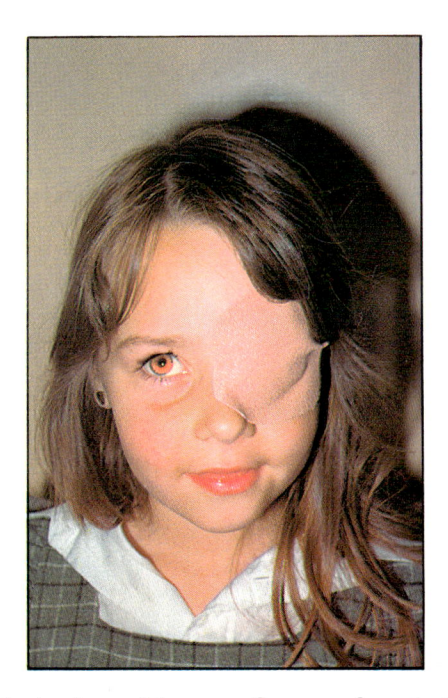

Figure 9.2 Occlusion. Sticking plaster is used to cover the normal eye in the treatment of amblyopia

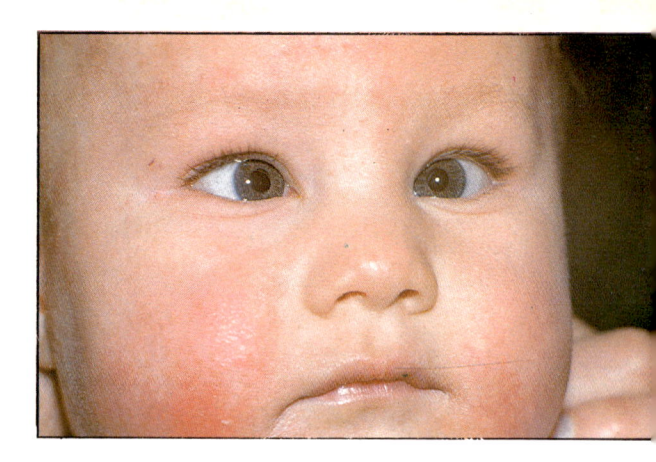

Figure 9.3 Right convergent squint. Displacement of the corneal light reflex to the temporal side of the right pupil is shown

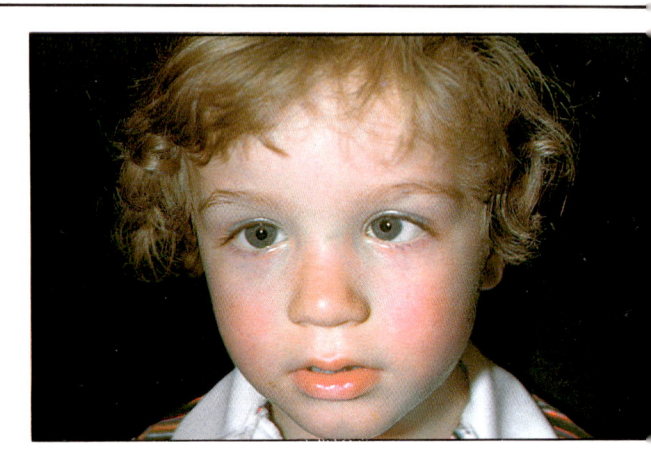

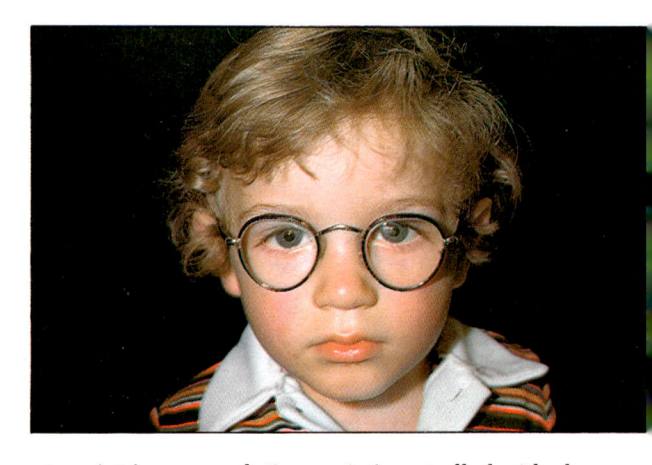

Figure 9.4a Left convergent squint (accommodative squint)

Figure 9.4b Left convergent squint (accommodative squint) controlled with glasses

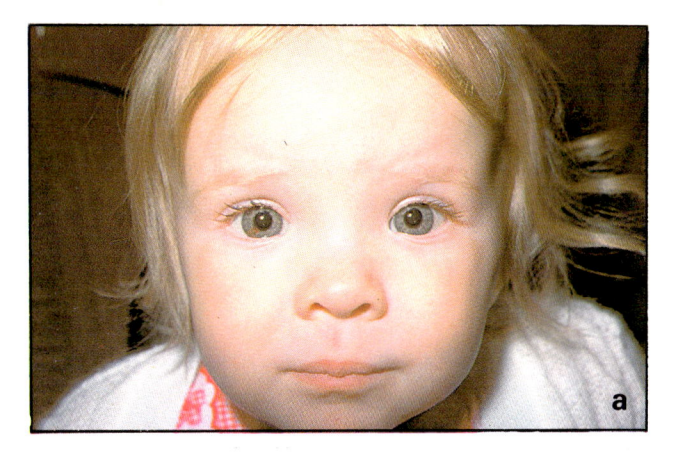

Figure 9.5a Epicanthus. There is no squint when the child is looking straight ahead

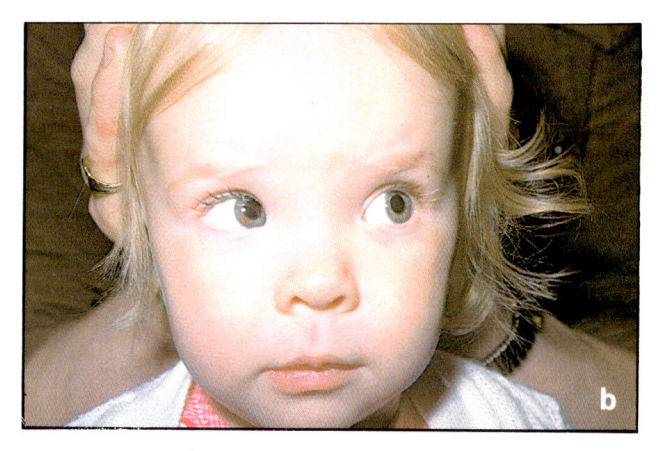

Figure 9.5b Epicanthus. There is an apparent right convergent squint when looking to the left

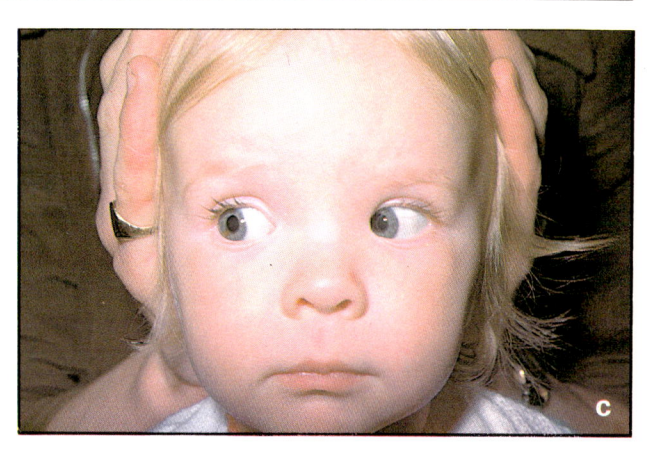

Figure 9.5c Epicanthus. There is an apparent left convergent squint when looking to the right

107

Figure 9.6 Ptosis

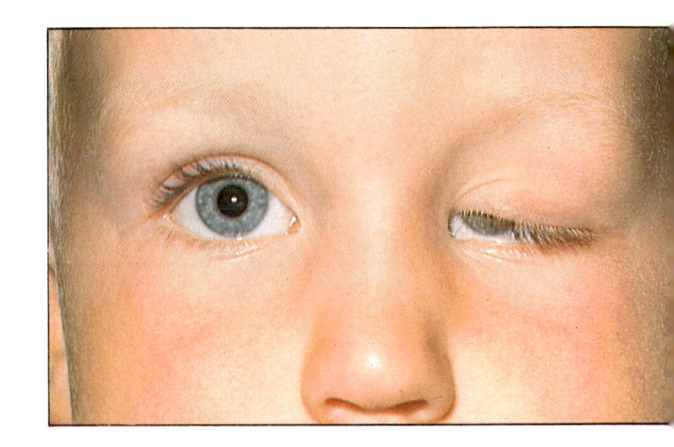

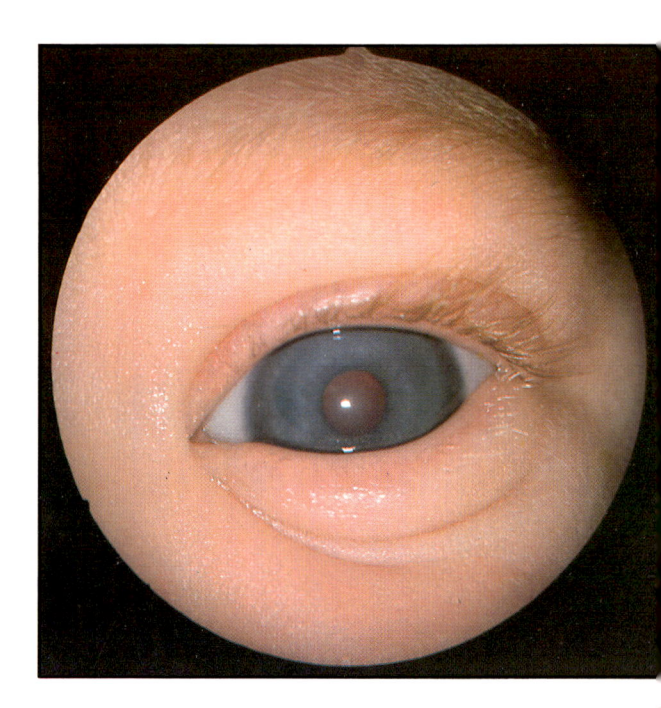

Figure 9.7 Congenital glaucoma: the enlarged hazy cornea of an eye with marked photophobia, blepharospasm and epiphora

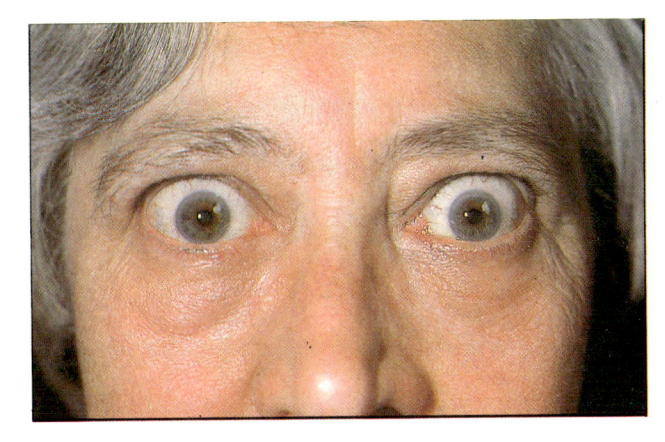

Figure 10.1 Thyroid eye disease. Upper lid retraction with fullness of the upper lids

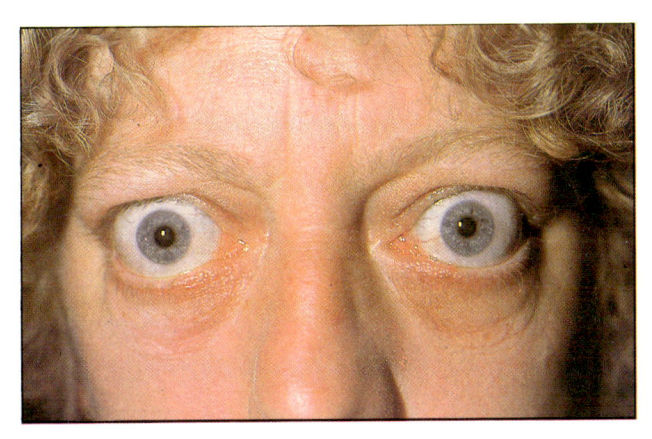

Figure 10.2 Thyroid eye disease. Upper and lower lid retraction with exophthalmos

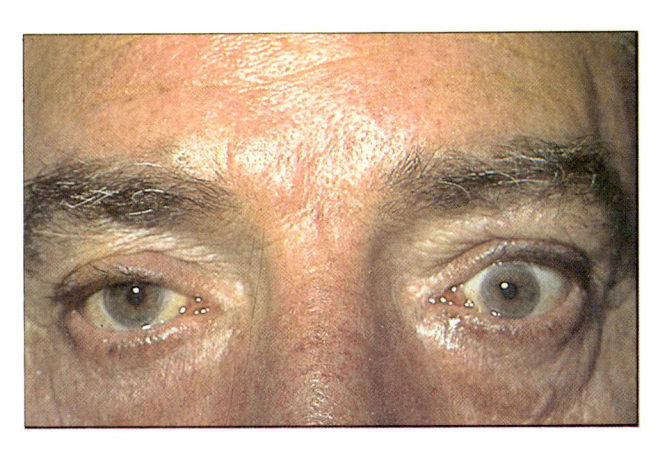

Figure 10.3 Thyroid eye disease. Unilateral lid retraction

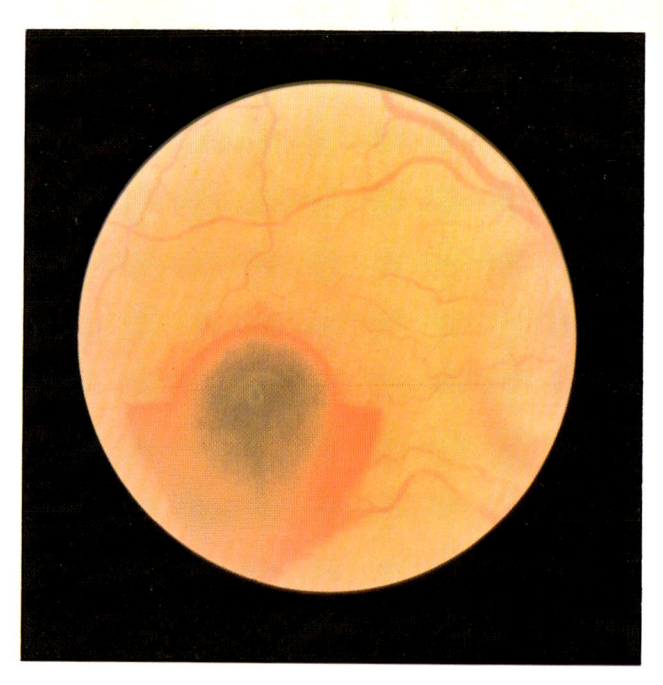

Figure 10.4 Subhyaloid haemorrhage with the typical straight horizontal upper border

Figure 10.5 Hypertension. Flame-shaped haemorrhages adjacent to a swollen optic disc

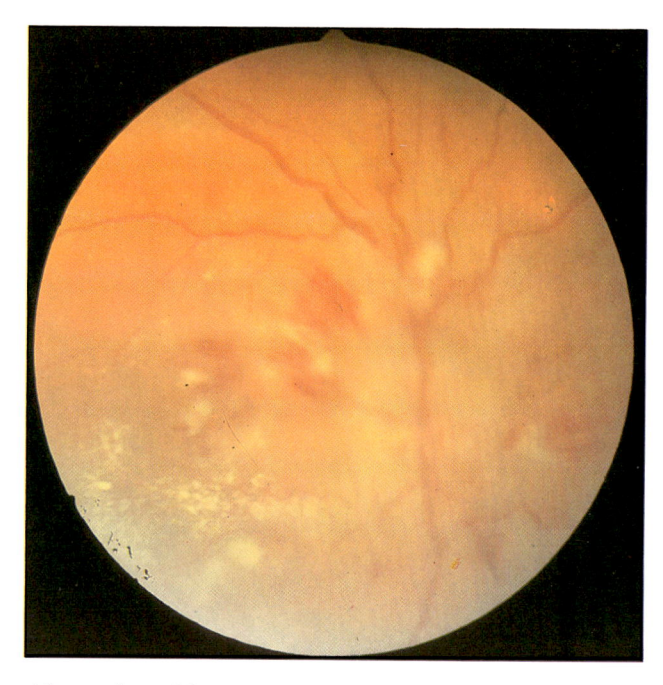

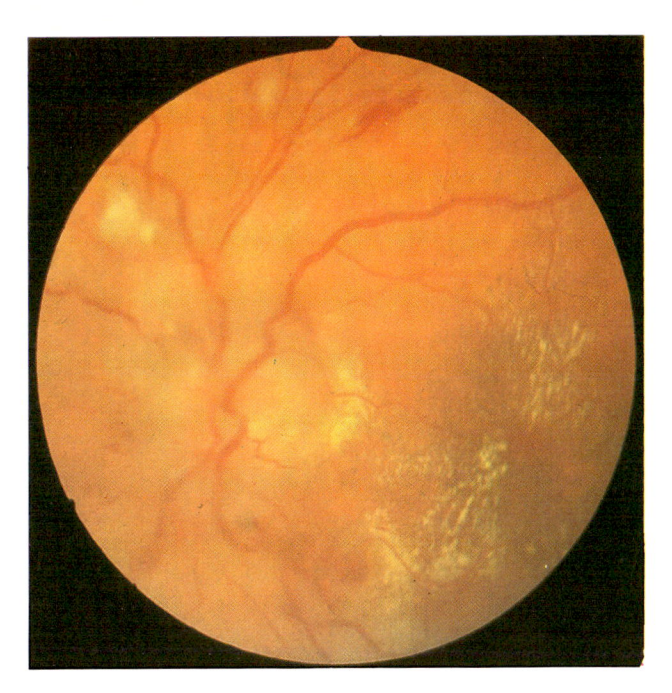

Figure 10.6 Hypertension. Hard exudates arranged in a macular star, scattered soft exudates and flame-shaped haemorrhages around a swollen disc

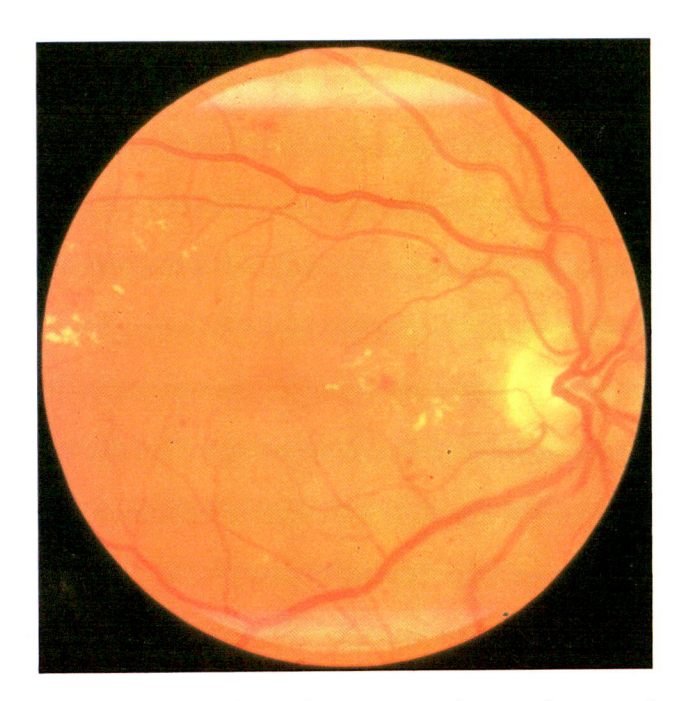

Figure 10.7 Diabetes. Background retinopathy with aneurysms, haemorrhages and exudates

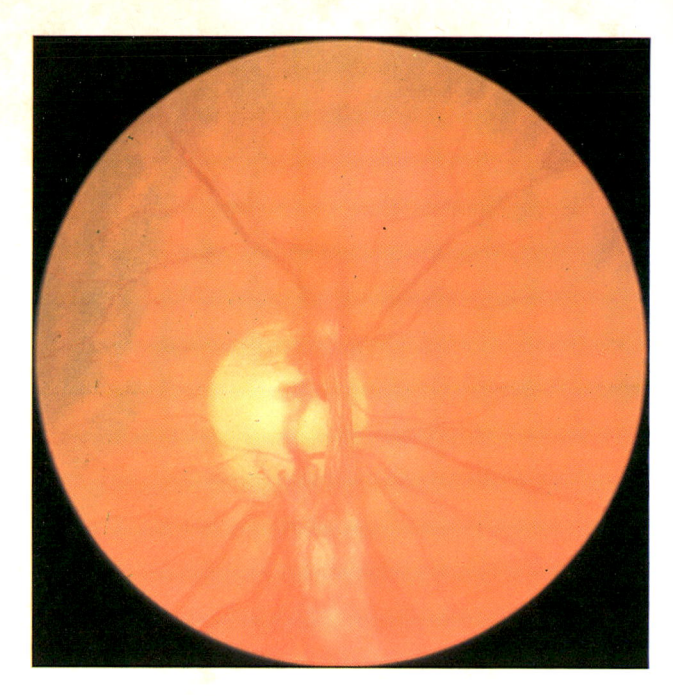

Figure 10.8 Diabetes. Proliferative retinopathy with neovascularization and a traction retinal detachment

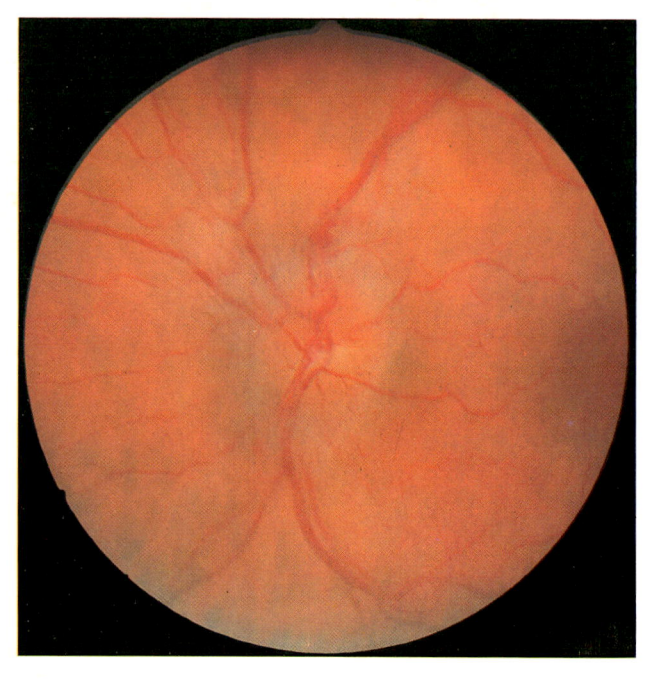

Figure 10.9 Papilloedema. Acute papilloedema with blurring of disc margin, hyperaemia, and venous engorgement

⑨ Paediatric ophthalmology

Introduction – Squint – Watering eyes – Ptosis – Congenital glaucoma – Retinoblastoma

Introduction

Childhood ailments usually result in parents seeking early medical attention, but occasionally misplaced advice from friends or relatives can delay the start of treatment. Such delay may be of no consequence if the problem is only a watering eye, but can result in a permanently lazy eye if a squint is present or may even be fatal if a retinoblastoma remains untreated.

Squint

Definition

The term squint is used to describe any abnormal deviation of the eyes. Numerous terms (cast, turn, cross-eyed) may be applied, so it is important to ask the parents to describe exactly what they have noticed.

Types of squint

The squint may be convergent with one eye turned inwards, divergent with one eye turned outwards or vertical when one eye appears higher than its fellow (**Figure 9.3**, p. 106). In all cases only one eye (the squinting eye) is deviated while the other (the fixing eye) looks straight ahead.

A paralytic squint is caused by weakness of an extraocular muscle, but this is relatively uncommon in children.

A non-paralytic squint has the same angle of deviation in all directions of gaze and is also called a concomitant squint.

Constant or intermittent

The squint may be constant or may be present only intermittently when the child is tired or ill.

Problems in ophthalmology

In near or distance vision It may be present when the eyes are used for close work or may only appear if the child is looking into the distance.

Family history There may be a strong hereditary factor with a family history of squint. This has particular relevance in those intermittent cases which only seem to be visible to the parents, but never in the doctor's surgery.

Diagnosis The presence of a squint may be obvious with the squinting eye markedly deviated. For smaller degrees of squint it is necessary to use the cover test (for details see Chapter 2, Examination).

Management All squints should be referred to an ophthalmic department. The 'wait and see' policy which is sometimes adopted may lose precious time for possible treatment. No child is too young to refer and children do not grow out of squints.

Aims of treatment The aims of treatment are to produce equal vision and normal co-ordination between the two eyes.

Vision The level of vision can be gauged even in very young children who do not know their letters.

The E test uses a cube with different sizes of the letter E which can be held in different directions. The child is encouraged to hold a cut-out 'E' in the same direction.

The Sheridan Gardiner test uses individual letters of varying size held by the examiner which are matched by the child on a separate card (**Figure 9.1**, p. 105).

All children are tested by an atropine refraction, which not only dilates the pupil, but also temporarily paralyses accommodation. This allows assessment of the refractive power of the eye and a chance to examine and exclude any other conditions affecting the retina or optic disc.

Atropine ointment is instilled into both eyes three times each day for 3 days before the test. The pupils remain dilated and the vision blurred for about 7–10 days while the effects of the ointment wear off.

Spectacles Spectacles are ordered if there is a focussing error that is large enough to prevent clear vision. It is possible for children to wear glasses from the age of 18 months, although accustoming them to this requires considerable patience and perseverance by the parents.

At birth the eye is only three quarters of the adult size and is hypermetropic, clear vision being achieved by accommodation. Accommodation and convergence of the eyes are closely linked and excessive accommodation in hypermetropia may result in overconvergence of the eyes. This convergent squint occurs with close focussing, and is called an accommodative

Paediatric ophthalmology

squint, and may be controlled with glasses (**Figure 9.4a & b**, p. 106).

Amblyopia   If the vision in one eye is weaker (amblyopia) despite a spectacle correction, patching or occlusion may be needed. By covering the normal eye the child is made to use the amblyopic eye.

Occlusion   Improvement in the vision can be achieved up to the age of 8 years, but thereafter the visual acuity is 'fixed'. The earlier that amblyopia can be treated, the greater the chance of improving the vision.

The eye is covered by applying sticking plaster to the spectacles or directly to the face (**Figure 9.2**, p. 105). This patch is worn for varying lengths of time under the supervision of an orthoptic department.

It is essential that the parents should understand the reason for patching, since their role in encouraging the child is so important. The stigma of a patch to a child of school age is often the cause of failure unless there is adequate family support.

Surgery   Surgical correction is necessary if spectacles fail to control a squint. For a convergent squint the medial rectus muscle is weakened (by recession) and the lateral rectus muscle is strengthened (by resection). The procedure is reversed for a divergent squint.

Two thirds of cases are straightened by one operation, but the remainder require further surgery particularly if there is a vertical element to the squint.

Anaesthesia   Surgery is performed under general anaesthesia and the child must be fit. During the winter months many unsuitable children are brought for surgery with an overt cold or the after-effects of one. If there is any doubt about the fitness for anaesthesia the operation should be postponed.

Some centres perform squint surgery as day cases while others admit the child for one or two nights.

Postoperative management   After operation a corticosteroid/antibiotic ointment (chloromycetin–hydrocortisone) can be given for 2 weeks. Spectacles should be worn unless a specific contrary order has been given.

The eye will remain red for 6 weeks, but normal schooling can be restarted after 1 week. Swimming should be avoided until any inflammation has settled.

Occasionally swelling may occur over a resected muscle due to the formation of a granuloma. This responds to local corticosteroid drops.

Problems in ophthalmology

Latent squint
    Most people have a tendency to squint, but it is controlled by the fusion in the brain of the two retinal images. This is a latent squint or heterophoria.

Manifest squint
    If the muscles become fatigued or if the retinal image in one eye is poor the latent squint may become manifest. The patient may see double or may only be aware of a strained feeling as the muscles strive to keep the eyes correctly aligned.

Treatment
    Orthoptic treatment by exercises may control small deviations, but ultimately surgical correction becomes necessary.

Epicanthus
    Epicanthus is a common cause for referral for an apparent squint. It is due to a wide bridge of the nose and epicanthic folds. These folds of skin extend from the upper to the lower lids and tend to hide the sclera of the medial side of the eyes. They are frequently asymmetrical. When the eyes are turned there appears to be unequal movement as the eye turning towards the nose tends to disappear behind the skin fold (**Figure 9.5a, b & c**, p. 107).

Management
    These cases should be referred to an ophthalmic department so that a genuine squint can be excluded.

    No treatment is necessary for epicanthus and the parents should be reassured that with the normal growth of the face the appearance will gradually improve.

Watering eyes

Watering eyes in children usually present soon after birth and are caused by the failure of the normal development of the nasolachrymal duct.

    Secondary infection often supervenes.

Management
    Under the age of 6 months local antibiotic drops should be instilled if the discharge is purulent. Massage of the lachrymal sac by pressure over the medial end of the lids may be sufficient to open the duct.

    If the watering persists, syringing and probing under a general anaesthetic are performed. This procedure may need to be repeated.

Ptosis

Cause
    Drooping of the upper lid may be congenital in origin. It is usually due to a defect of the levator muscle of the lid and may be associated with superior rectus muscle weakness. It is usually unilateral (**Figure 9.6**, p. 108), but may occasionally affect both eyes.

Paediatric ophthalmology

Management
All cases should be referred for assessment because of the potential dangers if left untreated.

Surgical correction is indicated if the pupil is covered. This is necessary to prevent the development of amblyopia which will occur if a normal retinal image is not achieved.

When the ptosis is only slight and there is no evidence of amblyopia the problem is cosmetic. Surgery may be necessary, but is best deferred until the age of 4 or 5 years.

Congenital glaucoma

This is a rare form of glaucoma, but important to diagnose if blindness is to be prevented. It tends to affect males more than females and is bilateral.

Presentation
The earliest symptoms are photophobia and blepharospasm which together cause the child to screw up the eyes even in normal daylight. Excessive watering of the eyes is also present. As the intraocular pressure rises the eyes enlarge (buphthalmos) and the corneal diameter increases. Haziness of the cornea is produced by leakage of fluid through splits in the deeper layers (**Figure 9.7**, p. 108).

Management
Early referral for surgical drainage operation is essential to prevent damage to the optic disc from the raised intraocular pressure.

Retinoblastoma

This exceedingly rare tumour of the retina is important because of the fatal outcome if left untreated. The condition may be hereditary.

Presentation
The tumour may cause a squint when the macula is involved and for this reason all children with squints must have their fundi examined. The tumour appears as a whitish mass arising from the retina. It may be bilateral. As the tumour enlarges into the vitreous cavity a whitish reflex may be seen in the pupil.

Management
The tumour spreads rapidly and early treatment is essential. The mass may be difficult to differentiate from other causes of a white pupil such as retrolental fibroplasia, endophthalmitis or an organized vitreous haemorrhage. Small tumours may be treated with radiotherapy and photocoagulation, but enucleation is usually necessary.

10 The eye and systemic disease

Introduction – Thyroid disease – The fundus – Hypertension – Diabetes – Papilloedema – Multiple sclerosis

Introduction

Many systemic conditions involve the eyes. In some, such as thyroid dysfunction or hypertension, the eye signs often give the first indications of the disease while in others, such as diabetes, the ocular changes may be a late manifestation.

Subtle changes in the external appearance of the eyes can pass unnoticed by the patient or near relatives and it is often the occasional visitor or general practitioner who may first notice an alteration in the facial appearance.

Thyroid disease

Hyperthyroidism

Hyperthyroidism or Graves's disease is the commonest cause for an alteration of the appearance of the eyes. The signs to notice are:

Signs
(1) Lid retraction
(2) Lid swelling
(3) Conjunctival redness and swelling (chemosis)
(4) Exophthalmos (synonymous with proptosis)
(5) Weakness of eye muscles.

Lid retraction
When the eyes are looking straight ahead the upper lid usually covers the cornea by about 2 mm, while the lower lid

Problems in ophthalmology

should rest against the limbus (junction of cornea and sclera).

Upper lid retraction is present if the sclera is visible above the cornea (**Figure 10.1**, p. 109). Lower lid retraction is present when a rim of sclera is present below the cornea (**Figure 10.2**, p. 109).

Lid lag
Retraction of the upper lid may be associated with lid lag. This is recognized by a widening of the strip of sclera above the cornea as the patient is instructed to follow a pencil that is moved from above downwards. The upper lid tends to lag behind the movement of the eyeball so that more sclera is momentarily visible. The transient nature of this sign makes it slightly unreliable.

Lid swelling
Pitting oedema of the lids with redness of the skin may accompany bulging around the eyes. The increased orbital contents tend to push forward so that a fullness appears above the eyes especially over the medial ends of the upper lids (**Figure 10.1**).

Conjunctival swelling
The conjunctiva tends to become swollen and thickened. This is most marked over the lateral sclera where the redundant conjunctiva may be loose and rest in a fold on the edge of the lower lid. Occasionally fluid may collect beneath the conjunctiva, forming a blister which looks like a reddish-yellow coloured blob of jelly on the eye.

Exophthalmos
Forward displacement of the eyeball causes retraction of the lower lid (**Figure 10.2**). This is present in one third of cases of hyperthyroidism, and is due to the increase in the volume of orbital tissues due to a generalized infiltration by mucopolysaccharides and oedema. This process also involves the muscles, causing weakness and double vision.

Ophthalmoplegia
The muscle involvement affects mainly elevation due partly to weakness of the superior rectus muscle and also to fibrosis of the inferior rectus causing inability to look up.

Unilateral or bilateral
All the signs tend to be bilateral, but unilateral involvement may also be met. Indeed, thyroid dysfunction is the commonest cause of unilateral lid retraction or exophthalmos (**Figure 10.3**, p. 109).

Occasionally the ocular signs may be present when there is no clinical evidence of thyroid dysfunction. In these cases called ophthalmic Graves's disease the eye signs tend to affect only one eye. Their management is the same as for Graves's disease as a proportion may eventually develop classical hyperthyroidism.

Management of thyroid eye disease
Mild cases may require only supportive therapy with occasional drops (methylcellulose) for the minor conjunctival irritation.

The eye and systemic disease

The management of severe cases can be difficult. The complexity of the laboratory tests in thyroid dysfunction together with the potential ocular problems means that these cases should be under the combined supervision of an endocrine and an ophthalmic clinic.

Treatment may be suggested as follows.

Lid retraction may be lessened with guanethidine 5% drops; however, any irritation or redness of the conjunctiva may be made worse by this treatment.

Conjunctival chemosis. Methylcellulose drops can limit the symptoms of irritation, but local corticosteroid drops may also be required. Local antibiotic therapy may be necessary if infection is present.

Corneal involvement. The exposed position of the cornea may result in superficial punctate keratitis due to drying of the normal tear film. Ulceration may occur, particularly on the lower half of the cornea. This results from exposure at night when the lid does not cover the cornea completely. Local antibiotic ointment and padding will overcome the acute episode, but a lateral tarsorrhaphy to narrow the palpebral fissure is eventually necessary.

Ophthalmoplegia. Double vision is best avoided by occluding one eye with an eye patch. Surgical correction is usually postponed until there has been no further change in the muscle weakness for at least a year as the condition may improve spontaneously.

Exophthalmos. The increased orbital pressure may seriously damage the visual acuity by compressing the vascular supply to the optic nerve. Immediate treatment with systemic corticosteroids is needed to prevent permanent loss of vision. If, despite this treatment, the vision continues to fail, surgical decompression of the orbit is required. This is performed either through the maxillary sinus or through the roof of the orbit by the transfrontal approach.

Hypothyroidism

The eye complications in hypothyroidism tend to be less noticeable than the general signs of this condition. There is oedema of the lids with loss of the eyelashes. The loss of the outer third of the eyebrows also occurs, but this is an unreliable sign since it is also seen in many normal patients of the same middle-aged group.

The fundus

The fundus of the eye presents such an easy opportunity to examine part of the vascular tree that a large number of changes have been described. Some of these are the result of disease, while others represent part of the wide range of appearance of the normal ageing eye.

Attempts to classify and grade these changes are of little practical use and do not help in the day-to-day management of the diseases.

The changes of diagnostic and practical importance are:

(1) Vessel changes
(2) Haemorrhages
(3) Exudates.

The variations in these aspects are of value in the assessment of arteriosclerosis, diabetes and hypertension. The picture of the fundus may be complicated as any one or occasionally two – and in the elderly all three – conditions may be present at once.

Vessel changes

Diameter
In childhood the retinal arteries and veins are approximately the same diameter. With increasing age there is a gradual narrowing of the arterial blood column. This is due to a thickening of the vessel wall which at the same time becomes hardened (arteriosclerosis). This generalized narrowing is difficult to assess because it is gradual. If, however, very narrow arteries are seen in young patients it is indicative of hypertension. Segmental narrowing of the arteries may signify hypertension in the arteriosclerotic patient.

Arteriovenous crossing
The retinal arteries usually cross over the veins with the venous blood column visible through the shared common adventitia.

Thickening of the sheath may cause concealment or even narrowing of the vein. Deflection of the vein is a more marked change.

Light reflex
The appearance of the light reflection from the retinal arteries alters with changes in the vessel wall.

The term 'copper wiring' is said to indicate mild changes while 'silver wiring' is used to describe more advanced arterial thickening. Both terms are best avoided as they do not serve to differentiate those eyes with ageing changes from those with hypertension.

The eye and systemic disease

Vascular sheathing is likewise not indicative of any particular pathological process. The blood column may become obscured in the normal elderly eye, or when hypertension, diabetes or vasculitis are present.

Obstruction within the retinal arteries may result from emboli (see Chapter 5, amaurosis fugax).

Neovascularization
The growth of new vessels is usually in response to ischaemia of the retina. This may occur in diabetes or following venous occlusion. More rarely it is seen with vasculitis. The neovascularization may be limited to the retina or may extend forward into the vitreous.

The fine irregular vessels are very fragile and haemorrhages from them are common. Forward growth into the vitreous (retinitis proliferans) is accompanied by the formation of fibrous tissue, shrinkage of which can cause traction and detachment of the retina.

Haemorrhages

The appearance of haemorrhages depends on the anatomical site.

Subhyaloid haemorrhage
Subhyaloid haemorrhage can occur when blood leaks between the retina and vitreous. It is characterized by the presence of a fluid level with a straight horizontal upper border (**Figure 10.4**, p. 110). The causes are vascular disease (diabetes, hypertension) particularly when neovascularization is present.

Flame-shaped haemorrhage
Blood in the nerve fibre layer produces a superficial retinal haemorrhage with a linear or flame-shaped pattern. This is typical of hypertension or retinal vein occlusion.

Dot haemorrhages
When the blood is within the retina the pattern is more discrete, each haemorrhage being small and clearly defined. Diabetes and retinal vein occlusion are the commonest causes.

Exudates

Exudates are traditionally classified as either soft or hard.

Soft exudates
Soft exudates, also called 'cotton-wool spots', are not strictly exudative in origin. Each lesion is due to ischaemia producing an infarct of the retina. It appears as a greyish area which gradually becomes white. The lesions are scattered throughout the retina, and vary considerably in size.

Soft exudates may be found in many systemic conditions (hypertension, diabetes, anaemia and collagen diseases).

Problems in ophthalmology

Hard exudates
Hard exudates are formed by collections of lipid within retinal macrophages. They appear as either isolated or confluent yellow-white deposits, mainly concentrated at the posterior pole of the eye. Occasionally a complete ring may be formed around a leaking capillary (circinate retinopathy) or radiating lines from the macula may give the appearance of a star or a fan.

Hard exudates are typically found in diabetes, but they are also found in hypertension and local retinal vascular disease.

Hypertension

Presentation
Hypertension is an insidious condition and is usually found by chance either on routine medical assessment or when the patient attends for spectacles. Occasionally double vision from a nerve palsy – typically involving the sixth cranial nerve – or sudden loss of vision from a vitreous haemorrhage, or a vascular occlusion may be a presenting ocular symptom.

Fundus changes
The fundus changes depend on the age of the patient and the level of the blood pressure.

Vessel changes
In the young hypertensive patient there may be generalized narrowing of the retinal arteries.

Arteriovenous crossing changes are an unreliable index of hypertension as nearly half of all normotensive patients over the age of 60 show such changes.

Hypertensive retinopathy occurs when the diastolic pressure exceeds 120 mmHg. The changes that can be seen include haemorrhages, exudates and oedema of the optic disc.

Haemorrhages
Haemorrhages are usually the flame-shaped variety and found near the disc (**Figure 10.5**, p. 110). They increase with the severity of the condition.

Exudates
Exudates of both the soft and hard type may be present (**Figure 10.6**, p. 111). Soft exudates are of serious significance but hard exudates may be merely part of generalized arteriosclerosis.

Papilloedema
Oedema of the disc is a sign of malignant hypertension requiring urgent treatment (**Figure 10.5**). The degree of papilloedema is usually not as marked as with raised intracranial pressure. The disc margin may appear blurred and retinal oedema involving the macula may affect the visual acuity.

Results of treatment
Haemorrhages and soft exudates clear within a few weeks of starting successful treatment. Hard exudates may appear to increase during the first month and then take up to a year to

The eye and systemic disease

resolve. Papilloedema usually clears within a few weeks, but vessel changes are unaffected by treatment of hypertension.

Hypertensive treatment should be undertaken with caution when the patient also suffers from glaucoma. The sudden lowering of the blood pressure may impair the perfusion of the optic nerve head and precipitate drastic losses in the fields of vision. Therapy in such a patient should only be started if essential and only then after consultation with an ophthalmologist.

Diabetes

Whilst the retina is the commonest ocular structure to be involved in diabetes, the lens and the extraocular muscles may also be affected.

Lens Blurred distance vision due to increasing myopia can be a presenting symptom of diabetes. When treatment is started the reverse occurs and the patient becomes hypermetropic, so that reading may become difficult. Referral for a refraction for new spectacles should be deferred until satisfactory control of the condition has been achieved.

Extraocular muscles Sudden diplopia may result from weakness of the muscles supplied by the third or the sixth cranial nerves. Although often accompanied by a unilateral headache the condition usually resolves spontaneously over several months. The patient should be advised to cover one eye to overcome the double vision.

Retinopathy The development of diabetic retinopathy is related to the duration of the disease and not to its severity. The onset of the retinopathy may be delayed by good control of the diabetes, but after 20 years 60% of patients show retinal changes.

The retinal changes are of two types, the so-called background retinopathy and the proliferative retinopathy.

Background retinopathy The early changes of *background retinopathy* can only be seen with the pupil dilated. Minute red dots appear in the region
Aneurysms of the posterior pole with the development of aneurysms. If these rupture, small haemorrhages occur which may enlarge (**Figure**
Haemorrhages **10.7**, p. 111). Generally the larger the haemorrhage the more serious the disease.

Exudates Small discrete exudates also occur at the posterior pole. These tend to come and go over a period of months.

Management Lipid-lowering drugs to remove exudates serve only to improve the appearance of the retina and do nothing to alter the final visual acuity. The only indication for their use is when there is hyperlipidaemia with cholesterol over 300 mg/100 ml. If the vision is normal no treatment is needed.

Problems in ophthalmology

Proliferative retinopathy	Ideally all diabetics should have a retinal examination with the pupil dilated once a year, but this is not always feasible. The reason for the examination is to exclude the development of treatable proliferative retinopathy.
New vessels	Neovascularization is the hallmark of *proliferative diabetic retinopathy*. The new vessels develop within or on the surface of the retina, but eventually extend forward into the vitreous
Vitrous traction	(**Figure 10.8**, p. 112). Fibrosis and contraction of intra-vitreal vessels produces traction on the retina and causes retinal
Retinal detachment	detachment. Recurrent haemorrhage from the new vessels is the eventual cause of blindness.
Haemorrhage	Occasionally neovascularization starts at the disc and, untreated, this type tends to have a worse visual prognosis.
Management	The early recognition of this type of retinopathy is important since photocoagulation can limit its complications.

Photocoagulation can be achieved with light either from a xenon arc or from a laser. The light produces a small burn in the retina and results of this treatment can be very dramatic with complete regression of the neovascularization. Laser treatment has the advantage of being performed under local anaesthesia on an outpatient basis, but requires many follow-up visits.

When repeated vitreous haemorrhage has occurred it is possible to excise the diseased vitreous (vitrectomy) and restore some useful vision. This is dependent on the state of the retina which can be assessed by the use of ultrasound scans (**Figure 10.10a & b**, p. 126).

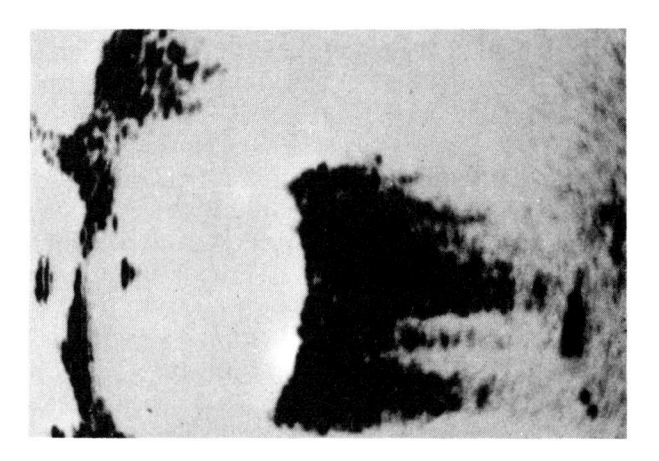

Figure 10.10a Ultrasound. Normal eye. (Courtesy M. Restori, Ultrasound Dept., Moorfields Eye Hospital)

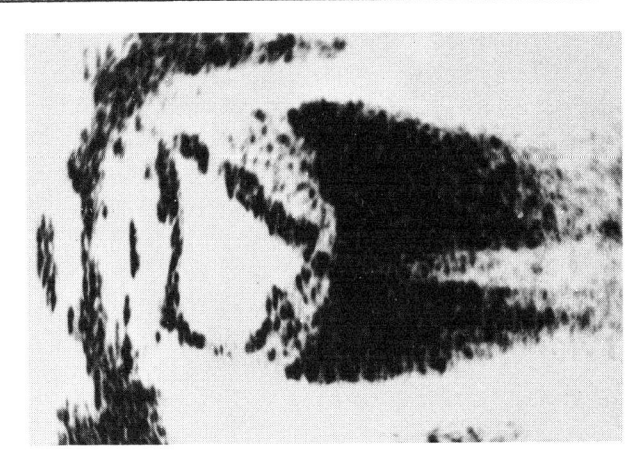

Figure 10.10b Ultrasound. Retinal detachment. (Courtesy M. Restori, Ultrasound Dept., Moorfields Eye Hospital)

Papilloedema

Acute

Chronic

Different-
iation from
papillitis

Management

Swelling of the disc occurs with raised intracranial pressure and malignant hypertension. The disc margin becomes blurred and the central physiological pit is filled in. Later the disc becomes hyperaemic and swollen and the retinal veins are dilated (**Figure 10.9a**, p. 112). Flame-shaped haemorrhages appear in the retina adjacent to the disc. When the swelling is gradual these acute signs may be absent and the disc becomes gradually pale. Papilloedema is usually bilateral. The visual acuity remains normal, although the blind spot is enlarged. The normal central vision helps to differentiate papilloedema from papillitis, in which the disc appears swollen and the visual acuity falls dramatically.

After hypertension has been excluded as a cause, all patients with suspected papilloedema should be referred to either an ophthalmologist or a neurologist.

Multiple sclerosis

Presentation

Age

Demyelination of the optic nerve with loss of central vision is a common presentation of multiple sclerosis. Tenderness behind the upper lid and pain on elevation precedes the attack by a few days. Involvement of the nerve supply to the extraocular muscles may cause weakness and result in diplopia.

The condition is commonest between the ages of 20 and 45, but rare after 60.

Problems in ophthalmology

Management
Recovery of the ocular problems is usually spontaneous over several weeks, but is not always complete. Treatment with corticotrophin, ACTH, may hasten the recovery, but has no effects on the long-term visual prognosis.

Although 50% of cases ultimately develop other signs of demyelination, these may be delayed for up to 20 years and may then be only minor and transient. It is, therefore, unjustified to disclose the suspected nature of the condition causing an isolated episode of retrobulbar neuritis, or diplopia.

11 Ocular pharmacology

Introduction

Most patients find that the application of any local drug to their eyes is difficult and slightly alarming. Advice from the doctor is often lacking as he may never have had to treat his own eyes. Effective treatment can only be expected if the correct drug is prescribed and the patient instructed in its proper application.

Ointment versus drops

Many eye preparations are available as ointments or in drop form.

Most patients find that eye drops are easier to use than ointment, which tends to remain on the nozzle of the tube rather than the eye, blurs the vision and usually makes the lids and face greasy. Eye drops are, however, rapidly eliminated from the conjunctival sac, whereas ointment remains and has a longer action. Systemic side-effects from absorption through the nasal mucosa or by ingestion occur more readily with drops than ointment.

Generally it is best to give eye drops by day and ointment by night.

Instillation of eye drops

The administration of eye drops is easier with the all-plastic containers than with the traditional glass bottle and pipette. The plastic containers are issued by the majority of proprietary manufacturers, but the glass bottle and pipettes are used by pharmacies for preparations which can be prepared in bulk to reduce costs. Most elderly patients prefer the plastic sort which do not spill and are easier to handle.

The method of drop instillation is as follows.

Problems in ophthalmology

(1) Pull down lower lid with forefinger of one hand holding the open bottle or pipette in the other hand.

(2) Move the bottle in front of the eye with the head tilted backwards.

(3) Look to the top of the head and squeeze the bottle at the same moment. The drop will then fall on the less sensitive sclera rather than the cornea. The bottle or pipette should not touch either the lids or the eye.

The manoeuvre may be easier if the patient lies on a bed, or sits with the head back in a chair.

Two drops will usually fill the conjunctival sac, and any excess will be blinked onto the lid margins. It is, therefore, impossible to instill too many eye drops.

Patients should be warned that they may taste the drops because of the normal tear drainage into the nose and onto the back of the tongue.

Instillation of ointment Ointment tends to be more difficult to administer. The method is as follows.

(1) Pull down the lower lid.

(2) Express about 5 mm (quarter inch) of ointment into the outer third of the lower fornix (the recess behind the lower lid).

(3) Close the lids to cut off the ointment from the tube. The tip of the tube is bound to touch the lids.

(4) Massage the eye gently to distribute the ointment and wipe any excess off the lids with a paper tissue.

All patients except the very young or the infirm should be encouraged to instill their own treatment. More regular therapy is then possible than if the patient is dependent on a relative or visiting nurse.

Sensitivity reaction Reactions to locally administered drugs are characterized by irritation and redness of the eyes and lids. Changes start within 36 hours of administration of the drug. The skin around the eyes becomes puffy and may develop an eczematous reaction. Later scaling occurs.

Changes may develop after starting a drug that has been successfully used on many occasions.

Causes The reaction may be a direct response to the drug or may be caused by the preservative in drops or the base in ointments.

Treatment The suspected medication should be stopped at once. The

Ocular pharmacology

skin of the lids and cheeks may be treated with a weak corticosteroid preparation such as hydrocortisone lotion (ointment and creams are difficult to apply to a weeping skin).

Corticosteroid eye drops (prednisolone or betamethasone) may be used, with caution, if the eye is severely affected. Local antibiotic eye drops may be needed if there is any infection, in which case corticosteroids should not be given.

Drugs in common use are listed in Table 11.1.

Table 11.1

Treatment	Generic name	Trade names United Kingdom	Trade names United States
Antibacterial	Chloramphenicol drops 0.5% ointment 1%	Chloromycetin Minims Sno-Phenicol	Chloroptic
	Gentamicin sulphate drops 0.3%	Genticin	Genoptic Garamycin
	Neomycin sulphate drops 0.5%	Minims Myciguent Nivemycin	
	Chlortetracycline hydrochloride 1%	Aureomycin	
	Tetracycline hydrochloride 1%	Achromycin	
	Sulphacetamide sodium drops 10%, 20%, 30% ointment 2.5%, 6%	Albucid Bleph-10 Liquifilm Isopto-Cetamide Minims	Bleph 10
Antiviral	Idoxuridine drops 0.1% ointment 0.5%	Dendrid Kerecid Idoxene Ophthalmadine	Stoxil
	Vidarabine ointment 3%	Vira-A	
	Trifluorothymidine drops 1%		Viroptic
	Acyclovir ointment 3%	Zovirax	
Anti-inflammatory: corticosteroids	Hydrocortisone acetate drops 1% ointment 2.5%	Hydrocortistab	
	Prednisolone sodium phosphate drops 0.5%	Predsol	

Problems in ophthalmology

Table 11.1 (continued)

Treatment	Generic name	Trade names United Kingdom	Trade names United States
	Betamethasone sodium phosphate drops 0.1% ointment 0.1%	Betnesol	
	Dexamethasone drops 0.1%	Maxidex	
	Fluorometholone drops 0.1%	F.M.L. Liquifilm	
	Clobetasone drops 0.1%	Eumovate	
Anti-inflammatory: Non-corticosteroids	Oxyphenbutazone ointment 10%	Tanderil	
	Sodium cromoglycate drops 2%	Opticrom	
Antiallergic	Xylometazoline hydrochloride + Antazoline sulphate	Otrivine-Antistin	
	Zinc sulphate + phenylephrine hydrochloride	Zincfrin	
Artificial tears	Hypromellose drops 0.1–1.0%	Isopto Plain Isopto Alkaline Tears Naturale	
	Polyvinyl alcohol drops 1.4%	Liquifilm Tears	Tears Plus
Glaucoma	Pilocarpine hydrochloride drops 0.5–4%	Isopto Carpine Sno-Pilo	
	Adrenaline drops 0.5–2%	Epifrin Eppy Isopto Epinal Simplene	
	Timolol Maleate drops 0.25%, 0.5%	Timoptol	Timoptic
	Guanethidine monosulphate drops 3–5%	Ganda Ismelin	
	Acetazolamide tablets 250 mg	Diamox	
	Dichlorphenamide tablets 50 mg	Daranide Oratrol	

Table 11.1 (continued)

Treatment	Generic name	Trade names United Kingdom	Trade names United States
Mydriatics	Cyclopentolate hydrochloride drops 0.5–1.0%	Mydrilate Minims	
	Homatropine hydrobromide drops 1–2%	Minims	
	Atropine sulphate drops 0.5–2%	Isopto Atropine Minims	
	Tropicamide drops 0.5–1%	Mydriacyl Minims	
Anaesthesia	Amethocaine hydrochloride drops 0.5–1%	Minims	
	Lignocaine hydrochloride drops 4%	Xylocaine	
	Oxybuprocaine hydrochloride drops 0.4%	Minims	

Index

acetazolamide, in acute glaucoma 45, 132
acute glaucoma 45–6
  presentation 45
  signs 45
  treatment 45–6
adenovirus, in conjunctivitis 41
adrenaline, in chronic glaucoma 85, 132
allergic conjunctivitis 41
amaurosis fugax 61–2
  findings 61–2
  management 62
  presentation 61
amblyopia 115
anaesthesia, drugs for 133
anterior chamber hyphaema 102
anterior uveitis *see* iritis
antiallergic drugs 132
antibacterial drugs 131
anti-inflammatory drugs,
  corticosteroids 131–2
  non-corticosteroids 132
antiviral drugs 131
aphakia, correction of 71–2
  contact lenses 71
  intraocular implants 71–2
  spectacles 71
aqueous drainage 86
arc eye 104
arteriovenous crossing, in thyroid disease 122

blepharitis 47
  squamous 47
  treatment 47
  ulcerative 47
blind register benefits 97
blow out fracture 102
blunt injury 101–3
  anterior chamber hyphaema 102
  blow out fracture 102
  iris 102
  lens 102
  management 102
  retina 102–3

carbonic anhydrase inhibitors, in glaucoma 86
cataract 67–72
  definition 67
  correction of aphakia 71–2
  management 68–9
  presentation 67–8
  surgical treatment 70–1
  unilateral 69–70
chalazion 48
chemical injuries 103
  acid and alkali 103
  treatment 103
childhood squint 113–6
  diagnosis 114
  epicanthus 116
  latent 116
  management

Problems in ophthalmology

spectacles 114–5
surgery 115–6
vision 114–5
manifest 116
types 113–4
chloramphenicol 32, 43, 131
  in conjunctivitis 32
  in dendritic ulcer 43
chronic glaucoma
  association with systemic disease 82–3
  hereditary basis 10
  intraocular pressure 82
  management
    medical 85–6
    surgical 86
  presentation 72, 81
  visual field changes 81
colloid bodies *see* drusen
colour vision, tests for 22
congenital glaucoma 117
conjunctiva 15, 50–1, 101
  colour changes 15
  cysts 51
  inflammation of *see* conjunctivitis
  in thyroid disease 120
  lacerations 101
  pinguecala 51
  pterygium 51
  subconjunctival haemorrhage 50–1
conjunctivitis 31–2, 41–2
  allergic 41
  bacterial 32
  causes 31
  symptoms 31
  TRIC agents in 41
  vernal 41–2
  viral 32, 41
contact lenses
  for aphakia 71
  for cataract 69
convergence 25–6
cornea
  abrasion 100
  examination 26
  foreign bodies 99
  penetrating injuries 101
cover test 23, 114
cupped disc 81
cyclopentolate (Mydrialate) 28, 132
dendritic ulcer 43
  presentation 43
  treatment 43
diabetes, ocular effects 82, 125–6
  extraocular muscles 125
  glaucoma and 82
  lens 125
  management 125–6
  retinopathy 125
disc 54, 72, 81
  cupped 81
  hypermetropic 54
  myopic 54
  normal 54, 72
discharge
  mucoid 14
  purient 14
  serous 14
  tears 14
disciform keratitis 43
dot haemorrhage 123
drusen 56

eclipse burn 104
ectropien
  cause 49
  treatment 49
endothelium 27
enophthalmos 15
entropion
  cause 49
  treatment 49
epicanthus 116
episcleritis
  symptoms and signs 42
  treatment 42
epithelium 26
E test 114
examination 17–29
  colour vision 22
  conclusions 29
  equipment 17
  external *see* external examination
  internal *see* internal examination
  visual acuity *see* visual acuity
  visual fields *see* visual fields
exophthalmos 120, 121
external examination 22–7

Index

convergence 25-26
cornea 26
  endothelium 27
  epithelium 26
  eyeballs 23
  eyelids 23, 26
  facial symmetry 22
  muscle weakness 22
  ocular movements 23
  pupil reactions 25
  skin changes 22
  squint *see* squint
  stroma 26-27
external eye 47-51
  conjunctiva *see* conjunctiva
  eyelid *see* eyelids
extracapsular extraction 70
exudates 123-4
  in hypertension 124
  in thyroid disease 123-4
eyeballs
  appearance 15
  position 23
eyedrops, instillation 129-30
eyelids
  appearance 14-5
  blepharitis *see* blepharitis
  chalazion 48
  ectropion *see* ectropion
  entropion *see* entropion
  eversion 26
  herpes zoster ophthalmicus *see* herpes zoster ophthalmicus
  normal position 23
  ptosis *see* ptosis
  retraction 23
  stye 48
  tumours of *see* eyelid tumours
eyelid tumours 49-50
  clear cyst 50
  papillomata 50
  rodent ulcer 50
  sebaceous cyst 50
  xanthelasma 50

facial symmetry 22
flame shaped haemorrhage 123
fleeting blindness *see* amaurosis fugax
floaters 53, 65
fundus
  appearance 53-4
  in hypertension 124
  in thyroid disease 122-4

giant cell arteritis *see* temporal arteritis
glaucoma
  acute *see* acute glaucoma
  chronic *see* chronic glaucoma
  congenital 117
  drugs for 132
guanethidine, in chronic glaucoma 85, 132

haemorrhages
  in blunt injury 102-3
  in diabetes 125, 126
  in hypertension 124
  in thyroid disease 123
  vitreous 64-5
herpes simplex
  in dendritic ulcer 43
  in follicular conjunctivitis 41
herper zoster ophthalmicus 48-9
  early symptoms 48
  eye involvement 48-9
  rash 48
  treatment 49
hypertension 124-5
  exudates 124
  fundus changes 124
  haemorrhages 124
  papilloedema 124
  treatment 124-5
  vessel changes 124
hyperthyroidism, ocular effects 119-21
  conjunctival swelling 120, 121
  exophthalmos 120, 121
  lid retraction 119-20, 121
  lid swelling 120
  management 120-1
  ophthalmoplegia 120, 121
hypothyroidism, ocular effects 121

internal examination 27-9
  anterior chamber 27
  intraocular pressure 29
  lens 27
  long sight 27

ophthalmology see
  ophthalmology
short sight 27
internal eye 53-7
  disc see disc
  floaters 53
  fundus 53
  macula 54
  opaque nerve fibres 57
  pigment see pigment
  retinal vessels 54
  toxocara 57
  toxoplasmosis see
    toxoplasmosis
  vitreous 53
intracapsular extraction 70
intraocular foreign bodies, X-ray
    for 101
intraocular implants 71-2
intraocular pressure
  assessment 29
  increase in glaucoma 45, 82
iridectomy 45-6
iridocyclitis see iritis
iritis 43-4
  cause 43-4
  presentation 44
  treatment 44

keratitis 42-3
  causes 43
  dendritic ulcer
    presentation 43
    treatment 43

lacerations 100-1
  conjunctiva 101
  skin 100-1
latent squint 23, 116
lens
  blunt injury 102
  examination 27
light reflex, in thyroid disease
    122-3

macula
  appearance 54
  degeneration see macula
    degeneration
macular degeneration 86-88
  disciform degeneration 87
  management 87-8

presentation 86-7
malignant melanoma 55
  findings 55
  treatment 55
manifest squint 23, 116
medical history 9-15
  family history 12
  general health 9-10
  previous ocular disease 9
  symptoms see symptoms
migraine 60-1
  management 60-1
  presentation 60
  visual aura 60
multiple sclerosis, ocular effects
    127-8
  management 128
  presentation 127
muscle weakness 22
mydriasis
  for ophthalmoscopy 28
  traumatic 102
mydriatics 132-3

naevus 55
near vision, measurement 21
neovascularization, in thyroid
    disease 123
non-contact tonometer 83

ocular movements, with squint
    23-4
ointment
  instillation 130
  versus drops 129
opaque nerve fibres 57
ophthalmoplegia 60, 120, 121
  in thyroid disease 120, 121
  migraine 60
ophthalmoscopy 27-9
  choice of instrument 27
  method 28-9
  pupil dilation 28

paediatric ophthalmology
    113-7
  congenital glaucoma 117
  ptosis 116-7
  retinoblastoma 117
  squint see childhood squint
  watering eyes 116
pain

Index

deep 13
referred 13-4
superficial 13
papilloedema 127
  acute 127
  chronic 127
  management 127
papillomata 50
partially sighted register benefits 97
penetrating injuries 101
  cornea and sclera 101
  X-ray 101
pharmacology 129-33
  drugs in common use 131-3
  eyedrops *see* eyedrops
  ointment *see* ointment
  sensitivity reaction 130-1
photophobia
  in iritis 44
  occurrence 13-14
pigment 55-6
  clumps 55
  drusen 56
  malignant melanoma *see* malignant melanoma
pilocarpine
  in acute glaucoma 45
  in chronic glaucoma 85
pinguecula 51
pinhole test 19-21
proliferative diabetic retinopathy 126
proptosis 15
pterygium 51
ptosis 14, 23, 116-17
  description 14, 23
  in childhood 116-17
pupil reactions 25
  consensual 25
  direct 25
  near reflex 25

radiation injuries 103-4
  infrared 104
  ultraviolet 104
red eye 31-46
  acute glaucoma *see* acute glaucoma
  causes 31
  conjunctivitis *see* conjunctivitis
  episcleritis *see* episcleritis
  keratitis *see* keratitis
  iritis *see* iritis
registration, of blind patients 88, 97
retina
  blunt injury 102-3
  detachment *see* retinal detachment
  vessels *see* retinal vessels
retinal artery occlusion 62
  findings 62
  management 62
  presentation 62
retinal detachment 65-6, 103
  findings 65
  from blunt injury 103
  management 65-6
  presentation 65
retinal vein occlusion 63-4
  findings 63-4
  management 64
  presentation 63
retinal vessels
  appearance 54
  occlusion 62, 63-4
retinoblastoma 117
  management 117
  presentation 117
retinopathy 125-6
  background 125
  proliferative diabetic 126
rodent ulcer 50
  presentation 50
  treatment 50

sclera
  colour changes 15
  penetrating injuries 101
sebaceous cyst 50
senile macular degeneration *see* senile macular degeneration
sensitivity reaction, to drugs 130-1
Sheridan Gardiner test 114
skin changes 22
Snellen chart 17-19
snow blindness 104
spectacles
  for aphakia 71
  for cataract 68, 69
  for squint 114-15
squamous blepharitis 47

Problems in ophthalmology

squint
  cover test 23
  family history 10
  latent 23
  manifest 23
  paediatric *see* childhood squint
  paralytic 23–4
Staphylococcus aureus 32
steroids, and dendritic ulcer 43
stroma, examination 26–7
stye 48
subconjunctival haemorrhage 50–1
subhyaloid haemorrhage 123
superficial injuries 99–100
  corneal abrasion 100
  corneal foreign bodies 99–100
  recurrent erosion 100
  subtarsal foreign bodies 100
surgery
  cataract 70–1
  chronic glaucoma 86
  malignant melanoma 55
  retinal detachment 65–6
  squint 115
symptoms, of eye disease
  appearance 14–15
  sensation 13–14
  vision 10–12
systemic disease, involving the eye 119–28
  diabetes 125–6
  hypertension *see* hypertension
  multiple sclerosis 127–8
  papilloedema 127
  thyroid disease *see* thyroid disease
temporal arteritis 62–3
  management 63
  presentation 63
thyroid disease, ocular effects 119–24
  fundus
    exudates 123–4
    haemorrhage 123
    vessel changes 122–3
  hyperthyroidism *see* hyperthyroidism
  hypothyroidism 121
timoptol, in glaucoma 85–6
tonometry 82, 83

toxocara
  management 57
  presentation 57
toxoplasmosis
  findings 56
  management 56
  presentation 56
  treatment 56
trauma 99–104
  blunt injury 101–3
  chemical injuries 103
  lacerations 100–1
  penetrating injuries 101
  radiation injuries 103–4
  superficial injuries 99–100
traumatic mydriasis 102
TRIC agents, in conjunctivitis 41
tumours
  eyelid *see* eyelid tumours
  malignant melanoma *see* malignant melanoma
  retinoblastoma 117

ulcerative blepharitis 47
unilateral cataract 69–70

vernal conjunctivitis 41–2
vessel changes, in thyroid disease 122–3
  arteriovenous crossing 122
  diameter 122
  light reflex 122–3
  neovascularisation 123
vision
  medical history 10–12
  slow loss of 67–72, 81–8
    cataract *see* cataract
    chronic glaucoma *see* chronic glaucoma
    macular degeneration *see* macular degeneration
  sudden loss of 59–66
    amaurosis fugax 61–2
    migraine 60–1
    retinal artery occlusion 62
    retinal detachment 65–6
    retinal vein occlusion 63–4
    temporal arteritis 62–3
    vitreous haemorrhage 64
visual acuity, examination 17–21

Index

    method   19
    near vision   21
    pinhole test   19–21
    results   19
    Snellen chart   17–19
visual disturbance   11–12
visual fields
    changes in glaucoma   81
    confrontation method   21–2
    distance vision difficulty   21
    reading difficulty   21

vitreous   53
vitreous detachment   53
vitreous haemorrhage
    causes   64
    findings   64
    management   64

xanthelasma   50
X-ray, for intraocular foreign
    body   101